The Alchemy of Herbs - A Beginner's Guide: Healing Herbs to Know, Grow, and Use

Adidas Wilson

Published by Adidas Wilson, 2017.

While every precaution has been taken in the preparation of this book, the publisher assumes no responsibility for errors or omissions, or for damages resulting from the use of the information contained herein.

THE ALCHEMY OF HERBS - A BEGINNER'S GUIDE: HEALING HERBS TO KNOW, GROW, AND USE

First edition. November 6, 2017.

Copyright © 2017 Adidas Wilson.

ISBN: 978-1393721499

Written by Adidas Wilson.

Table of Contents

Introduction

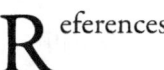eferences

Introduction

There is always something special about picking veggies and herb spices from your kitchen garden and enjoying their fresh nourishment. A small garden at the corner of your home can be exciting. Fortunately, growing herbs usually does not take up much space, whether you choose your balcony or the backyard. It is possible to find as much area as you need to bring the grocery right to your doorway.

Sunlight is the lifeblood of vegetation, and herbs are not an exception. It is thus important to assess the amount of sunlight your veggies can get at your selected location. Most need long hours of sunlight, up to six hours or so. However, some greens can do with less than this level. Yes, you might find yourself at crossroads with authorities or proprietor if your garden is in bear sight and too exposed that everyone can see it. Most importantly, you will need to consider another feasible location if the secluded backyard is not large enough for use. Timing is important if you want to get the best out of your garden. Not all seasons are similar, but it is worth timing and planting when you are certain the temperature are not likely to plunge to extremes. However, it is not always as strict as it may sound. If you have the right herbs on hand, you can take advantage of any temperature outside. And while the weather is so important, you can count on plants, potting soils, and pots among the most important essentials.

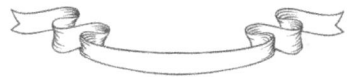

PROFESSIONALS ALWAYS have something to add virtually to anything we do, and taking care of your garden requires their services as much. Starting an herb garden is not as easy as it may seem, regardless of what you are planning on growing. Sprouting your tiny plants from scratch can be quite impressive and fun too. But if the space available is quite small, and the only time spurn for the season is not on your side either. Fortunately, you can get the best from the time available, if you can get sprouted greens from a nursery or farmers' market. Nevertheless, herb gardens are usually a promising endeavor, and a great way of ensuring a fresh and healthy recipe for your family.

Chapter 1

Grow Home Vegetables in your Backyard

S pending unnecessarily on a supermarket or grocery for fresh veggies, not to mention the last minute rush this can come with. Going this far is only an option, considering you can always pluck several fresh-from-the-garden leaves and enjoy the goodness of a homegrown recipe right from your backyard. Growing tender greens in your home garden is never as difficult endeavor as it may seem. It is simple, inexpensive and fun at the same time. And this is how it all begins;

The first step is shortlisting your favorite choices, especially the ones you use regularly. Starting with a few is always the best way to go as you learn the art of making veggies and watch them grow at the very front of your doorsteps. Once you are accustomed to the additional duty, you can now branch on to more options.

SELECT HERBS CAN GROW exceptionally well indoors or outdoors, in containers or the ground, it all boils down to what you want to do. If the space receives less than five hours of sunlight in a day, you might be better off going indoors for easier accessibility especially for watering and cooking. Besides, this helps prevent weeds, pests or fluctuating temperatures.

Seeds are quite cheap, but take longer and require more resources to grow. While on the other hand, seedlings are faster to grow, but only available in spring and summer.

Several gardening tools are essential, may be a spade, gloves, pots, containers, virtually anything you need for the job. And remember, some fertilized soil is important too, this can be naturally generated, or a general-purpose compost solution from a gardening store. For container gardening, a packaged potting soil mix can go a long way, as you will have little, to no worry about pests.

WHEN PLANTING SEEDS, consider starting with moist soil and covering with about half an inch of soil. It will take the seeds about a week to germinate. For potted seedlings, you can go for this process as well.

Watering is essential for your veggies, and applying water at the base of the plant whenever the soil dries a little can go a long way. Weeding is also necessary to prevent the unwelcome intruders stealing nutrients in the soil and competing with your greens. Now, if your greens are outside, bring them in before the onset of frost.

Harvesting is the time to get your reward after the hard work. Yet again, depending on what you want to get from your herbs, leaving a few leaves will mean others will grow. You can handpick the leaves or use shears.

After you have harvested your herbs, you can go for different methods of preservation, if you are not only using them. Taking care of your herbs from planning to harvest can seem to be quite a journey, but it is not as overwhelming as it seems. The fruits are sweet, and soon the process becomes more of a regular thing and fun as well.

Chapter 2

Imhotep and the Origin of Medicine

Greece was previously regarded as the origin of medicinal science; it has been proven that it all started with an Egyptian. Imhotep, also termed as the Prince of Peace, was the African genius who invented the art of medicine and healing. Imhotep supposedly received a book of healing from ancestral African forces, which was then given to the world and the foundation of modern medicine and surgery.

This pioneer was appreciated by the entire ancient world. Even the Greek's renowned Father of modern medicine, Hippocrates, celebrated this man of wisdom. According to scientists who have been scrutinizing documents as old as three centuries ago, ancient Egypt was the mother of modern medicine. The medical papyri studied by these scientists were written around 2,500 BC, about a century before the birth of Hippocrates.

Imhotep remains the world's first ever physician and first doctor, among other specifications as a priest, sage, poet, astrologer, and scribe to mention just a few. And more to it, he was an architect, credited for his building of Egypt's first pyramid. Imhotep is also believed to be the author of Edwin Smith Papyrus with over 48 described injuries and more than 90 anatomical terms. Besides, he founded a school of medicine in the area of Memphis, known to have existed for about two centuries.

Ancient Egyptian medical practitioners used honey, resins and antimicrobial elemental metals to treat wounds. Interestingly, this way of things is still practiced in the medical world to date. The most intriguing thing is that some of the remedies that Egyptian physicians prescribed were more than modern expectation. Such include saffron and celery, which were used for rheumatism are now at the heart of research on pharmaceutical field.

Moreover, pomegranate, which was used to fight tapeworms, has been used in clinical settings until the last five decades. Additionally, laxatives prescriptions included colocynth, castor oil. These are also used in our times for the same purposes.

Figs and bulk bran were used for promoting regularity, the same order that is done today in the medical arena. According to other references, as it is the case today, hyoscyamus was essential for treating colic. Coriander and cumin were useful as intestinal carminatives.

For musculoskeletal disorders, rubefacients were used to trigger blood flow as well as poultices, warming and soothing. The same is applied in modern times in sport medicine. Again, for cough remedy, Acacia is an essential solution, and aloes make the best solution for soothing and healing different skin conditions. The Egyptian physicians also came up with the use of essential oils and resins. Generally, about half of plants being used today were also used in ancient Egypt clinical setting.

Ancient Egyptian physicians were long forgotten as the origin practitioners of medicine. But despite this fact, it is safe to say that they were an essential part of the beginning of a new era of dealing with ailments. Considering that most of their practices are still in use today, it is obvious the sophistication of this medicine tech from centuries ago was a big breakthrough. Apparently, this knowledge will continue into the future of this essential field in society.

Chapter 3

St. John Wort & Depression

Plants have been an essential part of our medicine industry for centuries, and St. John wort is one of the most used ones. But as much as this plant is a renowned remedy for different health purposes, consumers need to understand some concerns about the safety and efficiency of the plant.

Also known as Hypericum perforatum, this plant has been widely used in Europe for thousands of years, dealing with mental conditions as well as depression. But according to the current evidence, this plant's effectiveness for depression are yet to be confirmed, not to mention that it has the potential for side effects as well. In the U.S. this plant has not been given the green light for use as an over-the-counter or prescription drug for depression.

Depression is primarily a medical condition that affects one in every ten adults in the United States. This can range from mood, thoughts, behavior and health. However, the severity of the condition and the symptoms thereof differ from one person to another. Conventional medicine can help in treating this problem, and these include psychotherapies and antidepressants.

As much as this plant has been used for centuries, it is known to affect the body's processing of a number of drugs, and is capable of causing colossal side effects.

Psychosis is unusual but possible side effect could result from taking St. John's wort. It is most likely to occur in people at a risk of mental health disorders like bipolar.

Serotonin is a brain chemical that antidepressants usually target, and as such, combine S.t John's wort with these drugs, and serotonin can increase to life-threatening levels. The result effect is known as serotonin syndrome. The symptoms of this condition can range from decreased body temperature, confusion, tremor and diarrhea, muscle stiffness, and sometimes death.

S.t John's wort is also known to suppress many prescription medicines. These include medicines like; antidepressants, digoxin (heart medication), cyclosporine (responsible for preventing rejection of transplanted organs by the body), and HIV drugs like indinavir. Others include drugs like warfarin and medications employed to thin blood, and several cancer medications like irinotecan. The other side effects are minor and uncommon, like upset stomach, or sensitivity to sunlight. If you are using this medication for depression, you will need to consider some things beforehand.

First, do not use it to replace conventional medical care for a medical problem, as in a case of depression, if not well treated, the situation might graduate to something severe. In such cases, seeking a healthcare professional is essential.

Keep dietary supplements in check, as these may cause medical problems if used incorrectly or over consumed, while others may interact with the medication with unpleasant effects. It is, thus, important to consult your healthcare provider.

And for pregnant women, nursing mothers and children, the situation is different, since many dietary supplements for these categories have not been tested. Besides, little is known about the effects that St John's wort could have on these groups of people, which calls for consulting your physician on the same.

St. John's wort has much to offer for the medicine industry, but it comes with a fair share of downsides as well. It seems the best way to get as much as possible out of this plant is knowing what to do and what to expect, and most importantly, work closely with your healthcare provider.

Chapter 4
Herbs in Small Spaces

The taste of fresh vegetables and fruits can be tantalizing. But this does not come easy; nevertheless, nothing can compare to the taste of freshly snipped veggies from your small garden near the house. The only problem is the usual lack of space to grow your herbs, especially if you are living in an apartment. But you can always make use of the insufficient space available and still make great veggies out of the space available.

If all you have beyond your door is nothing more than a balcony, containers will come to your rescue. The best thing about this method is that you can grow virtually any fruits or vegetables in your container gardening, especially if your container is the right size for the job. Besides, container gardening offers an opportunity for space saving as every single ounce of the soil in the container is important.

KEYHOLE GARDENING OFFER the best opportunity to maximize space, as there is no need for walkways like the case in most other garden types. The design here is simple; the bed is circular and high, with a "keyhole" access at the center for accessing the garden. The circle center has a vertical tunnel used for multiple layers of compost, which delivers moisture and nutrients as it breaks down. And above all, keyhole gardens are the go to option as they can be built using a variety of materials.

When it comes to vertical gardening, the list of opportunities is almost endless. Talk of conventional trellis, recycled pallet planter, hanging hydroponic window gardening, you name them. All need here is a little bit of creativity, and you are on the right track to an incredible herb gardening. Interestingly, as much as there is a vast number of ways to practice vertical gardening, the fruits and veggies you can choose from are as vast. From cucumbers to tomatoes, Asian greens and strawberries, peas and pole beans as well as kitchen herbs, there are a lot of options out there.

You can use square foot gardening with the raised beds model, and they are an ideal way to get the best space and minimize efforts. Raised beds not only offer space for more plants, but also require less need for weeding besides making it easier.

Now, now, now, what can be more than an edible landscaping, where you can replace ornamentals with fruitful greens? With the wide variety of edible ornaments around, you have every chance to turn the available space into a food source.

There is a lot you can do with a small space, provided you know what to do. Perhaps the best thing is that with these options at your disposal, getting the best out of every inch around is easier than it may sound.

Chapter 5
Remedies for HPV Virus

H uman Papillomavirus (HPV) is primarily an orgasm responsible for infections in humans, especially through genital contact during anal, oral or vaginal sex. The infection can also spread as a result of skin contact with an infected person, whether straight or same sex partner. Even worse, this might lead to juvenile-onset recurrent respiratory papillomatosis (JORRP), which happens in some cases where the virus can spread to a baby in case of a pregnant woman. HPV further has a darker side, as the infected person might not know about it, but this can be diagnosed through a series of symptoms.

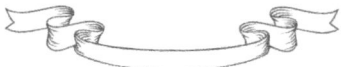

THESE INCLUDE DEVELOPING warts around the genitals, like the vagina and cervix. The same can also appear around the mouth or throat, and while there is virtually no cure for the infection, some natural ailments are being used to help people with the situation.

ECHINACEA, ALSO KNOWN as the purple coneflower, this is a perennial prairie herb, which is useful as tincture and tea. It offers an essential protection against warts, thanks to its phytosterol and polysaccharides that are important for improving the white blood cells that destroy the virus, therefore a reliable and natural remedy for this virus.

Goldenseal usually used alongside the Echinacea, this natural remedy for HPV is reliable for getting rid of warts. It is essential for triggering the immune system through increasing the amount of white blood cells. This plant has a twisted system known as rhizome, which comes in as a natural remedy. This is all thanks to its substance, berberine, since it bears a composition that kills strains in microorganisms.

CALENDULA IS ALSO KNOWN as a marigold flower. This is a natural method of treating HPV, usually consumed as a suppository or orally for treating warts. This plant's oils are effective for removing warts resulting from HPV infection.

Oregano oil, belonging to the mint family, this natural remedy acts by significantly reducing warts. To get the desired effect, this oil is to be applied directly to the wart itself, but make sure to dilute it. Curcurmin is an anti-oxidant, a purified form of turmeric that is effective in fighting HPV and protecting the body's DNA cells as a whole. Besides, it is essential in treating different types of cervical cancer.

Thuja leaf and oil of this herb have an antiviral element that helps fight HPV warts in the genital area by stimulating immune system cells that search and kill the virus-infected cells.

Pau D'Arco, the liquid extract of this plant offers a composition that fights the effects of the virus when applied on the region affected by the warts. It is efficient in shrinking them and getting rid of them completely. Mushrooms include Reishi and Shitake types of the mushrooms, a natural remedy for this virus infection. This is attributable to its antiviral activity that helps kill the virus' effects, hence depleting warts.

Tea tree oil is natural remedy for HPV with an antiviral and antimicrobial capability to diminish warts, the tea tree oil is a topical disinfectant with the ability of increasing the immunity level in the body.

Astragalus is also a natural agent that fights the virus by initiating the p53 gene that in turn stimulates interleukin-2 production, killing the virus as well as improving immunity against cancer. Garlic cloves have strong antimicrobial capability, not to mention its special substance called Allicin, which has the ability to destroy pathogens. You can apply it directly on the area with warts for relief. These are some of the most natural and effective solutions to deal with HPV virus, so you can go for whichever of them work best for you.

Chapter 6
Medicine Advanced from Ancient Societies

The field of medicine has developed over the centuries with new inventions and occasional technological advancements. But all this started somewhere, and the traditional means were so effective some of them are still in use today. So where did it all begin? Here is a brief history of the medicine industry over time.

In the early days, priests relied on rituals and other medical techniques in curing ailments. Sometimes, they could achieve greatness that could be carried on to future generations. Herbs, prayers, and acupuncture were among the methods used for healing. The Ancient Egyptians and Middle East were among the pioneers, and western practitioners played a vital role and took part in knowledge sharing.

In Egypt, herb-rich diet was essential for healthy builders of significant structures in the empire. They were usually well fed with a diet high in garlic, onion, and radish among others. Modern researchers have found these herbs to be highly rich in allicin, allistatin, and raphanin. These powerful natural antibiotics are essential for preventing disease outbreaks especially in crowded areas like work camps. What's more, practitioners in ancient Egypt were also renowned for their expertise in performing eye-surgery.

BESIDES, EGYPTIAN PHYSICIANS were also adept in suturing wounds as well as using raw meat to fasten the healing process as well as boosting blood production. Honey was also useful for its stimulation of secretions that aid infection-fighting white blood cells and its antiseptic qualities as well. And that's not all, priest-doctors also used molded bread for antibiotic purposes way before penicillin could be discovered by Alexander Fleming. Well, medicine was also practiced in Greece as well, and to an interesting extent for that matter.

To an extent, the Greeks believed in the power of prayers to the God of Medicine for healing. As such, many of the Greeks went to great temples for healing, making sacrifices and prayers to the god for their ailments to be healed. But Hippocrates' separation of the divine from the medicine contributed significantly to the history of this field.

To Hippocrates, studying the symptoms, giving diagnosis and eventual administration of treatment was the way to go. However, most Greeks considered combining the medicine process with the rituals performed by the priests. To the ancient Greeks, four humors applied to make up the body, in which if there were imbalances, mental as well as physical illnesses and ailments could be inevitable.

And these humors' balance would be founded on location, diet, age, and climate among other factors. The focus for the Greeks was to restore this balance.

Although the Roman's contribution in medicinal history is usually foregone, they served a crucial part as well. The only frequently recognized player is Galen, who was also of Greek origin, and who is considered to be worthy of mention.

But Romans had military surgeons who were adept in the art, offering procedures that guaranteed lower chances of deaths from infection. This was way beyond the success of other armies in saving lives through medicine-based care. As the empire split, the Western part lost its touch, but the Eastern one continued to perfect their skills. And this developed the knowledge that formed the basis for Islamic medicine.

Medicine has come a long way, from the historical eras from time immemorial. The pioneers of this art went far and wide to grow it over time, and the industry is still growing since then. The preservation of documentation of the history of medicine points out the footprints of the industry for historians.

Chapter 7
History of Ayurvedic Medicine

Ayurvedic medicine originated from the Indian subcontinent, spread across the globe and has been modernized over time. The tradition is basically a type of alternative medicine, with the Ayurveda therapies and practices travelled into the Western world.

This is believed to be god's gift to mankind through Hindu god, Ayurveda, who incarnated himself as a king of Varanasi, then taught medicine to a group of physicians. Some researchers consider Ayurveda as pseudoscientific, but others take it for a protoscience. Almost 21% of the Ayurveda medicine sold online by U.S and India manufacturers was found to be toxic with heavy metals like arsenic, lead and mercury. In India, the challenge of metallic contaminants on health is apparent.

Some of the medicine's concepts are said to have been around since the Indus Valley Civilization, with Ayurveda developing significantly during the Vedic period. But later, some of the non-Vedic period systems like Buddhism and Jainism developing some medical concepts as well as practices seen in most Ayurveda texts. According to the earliest Sanskrit, medical science is divided into eight major components;

These include the following;

General medicine (medicine of the body)

Dealing with spirits and possessed persons

Treatment of children (pediatrics)

Surgical ideas and removal of foreign objects,

Toxicology

The theoretical ideas of Ayurveda started around the mid-first millennium BCE. However, they differ from Buddhism and Jainism, as well as Samkhya and Vaisheshika philosophies. However, balance is stressed while suppressing natural urges is believed to cause illnesses. It is also advisable to uphold balance and measure when in pursuit of natural urges. Such include sexual intercourse, food and sleep intake. Besides, humoral balance is as important

Ayurveda further points out three significant substances. These are doshas, also known as Vata, Kapha, and Pitta. It also states that balancing the doshas brings health, and an imbalance leads to disease. By the medieval period, practitioners of this medicine had already developed several surgical procedures and medicinal preparations.

According to Ayurveda practitioners, mental existence, physical existence and personality are a single unit, and each of them has the potential of influencing the others. This is one of the fundamental aspects of Ayurveda, and an approach employed in diagnosis and therapies. Besides, Ayurveda has yet another part, which purports the existence of channels known as srotas for transporting fluids, which can be opened with the use of massage treatment. This treatment involves the use of oils and Swedana, but on the other hand, unhealthy channels are believed to cause diseases.

Diagnosis of illnesses in Ayurveda is based on eight things. These include Mootra (urine), Nadi (pulse), Jihva (tongue), Mala (stool), Sparsha (touch), Druk (vision), Shabda (speech) and Aakruti (appearance). Practitioners of this medicine major on the use of five senses like heating, used for observing condition of speech and breathing.

Most Ayurveda substances are based on plants, like the roots, leaves barks and fruits. Sometimes, seeds like cardamom and cinnamon are also used. In the 19th century, authors summarized hundreds of medicines derived from plants and their uses. These also included microscopic structures, toxicology, chemical composition, and other aspects documented. Ayurveda is not only based on plant products, animal ones such as bones, milk and gallstones are also useful.

Ayurveda has survived a long time in the medicine industry, and seems to be headed to more appreciation in the future. This can be attributed to the medicine's uniqueness and efficiency among others, but today's world development is apparently taking over this age-old medicine

Chapter 8

Traditional Chinese Medicine

O ver several decades, Eastern alternative (also called complementary or integrative) medicine practices have been implemented into healthcare facilities in the U.S. as well as other Western countries. The TCM herbs and therapies come with an extreme amount of benefits that has seen these types of medicine become recognized in the medicine world.

A study conducted in 2013 by Health Products Research showed that over half of U.S. physicians were planning to increase or start using alternative medicines. These include the renowned Traditional Chinese Medicine (TCM) within the course of the consecutive year.

Apparently, an ever-increasing number of medical schools are realizing and recognizing the necessity of including "mind-body" aspects in training their students and staff. These practices are inclined towards the importance of disease prevention as well as holistic treatments. Most patients and physicians usually question the effectiveness of TCM. But research has continuously showed that such complementary modalities can bring out significant differences in most of patient lives.

TCM stands for Traditional Chinese Medicine; is a holistic and natural health care system that has been around for two centuries, dating back to the year 200 B.C. The "holistic" and "natural" essence of TCM comes from the fact that it stimulates a mechanism that helps the body heal itself. More importantly, rather than merely depending on several apparent signs or symptoms, it involves every aspect of a patient's life.

In TCM, the body is considered to be a network formed by complex interconnected parts (also known as QI) and not as isolated organs or systems.

The kidney, liver, heart, gallbladder, lung, large intestines, small intestines, and liver are the most significant organs for TCM treatment. The benefits of TCM vary considerably, depending on the specific type used. This form of medicine is recognized as useful for treating multiple types of health problems.

Chinese herbal medicine is considered to be a major aspect of Traditional Chinese Medicine, and has been in use in China for centuries. It should also be remembered that herbs are highly ranked as essential for fundamental therapy used for treating numerous chronic illnesses as well as acute problems. One of the most recognized parts of this medicine, Chinese herbal therapy, comes from a traditional medicine text known as "Materia Medica." Trained herbalists use different minerals, teas, herbs, tinctures and several other extracts under this category. Any of these are used depending on the symptoms seen in a patient.

TCM comes with numerous benefits, from, reducing chronic headaches and chronic pain to lowering inflammation to increasing cancer protection. It is also essential for balancing hormones and improving fertility. Furthermore, it is important for liver health, and protecting cognitive health. TCM medicine further offers unprecedented effect in lowering stress response in the body, preserving muscle strength, balance and flexibility.

Considering the effectiveness of TCM and the related herbal therapies, it is obvious this form of medicine is worth the recognition in the medicinal industry across the globe. And with the advances of technology, it is possible that this tradition has a lot to offer. Only time will tell as to how much can be achieved from the use of this medicine.

Chapter 9
Cancer & Herbs

Cancer has been one of the biggest threats to the modern world. Unfortunately, most people are losing their lives to this menace despite the efforts by the medical industry to curb it. And it seems the natural solutions are becoming more promising.

Frankincense oil therapy was recommended by Dr. Budwig in cases like fighting brain tumors has seen considerable success. The method is being put to the test by researchers in trying to identify its cancer-fighting abilities. And the Indian frankincense has been proved to have a potential effect on treating cancers like; Breast, colon, prostate, brain, stomach (7 to 11), and pancreatic cancer.

Gerson therapy & juicing treatment was developed over ninety years ago by Dr. Max Gerson. He helped hundreds of people suffering from cancer activate an extraordinary ability in their bodies to heal itself through several ways like using; raw juice, organic-based foods, coffee enemas, natural supplements and beef liver among others in their diet. This treatment comprises mainly of the Gerson diet, juicing and detoxification.

Protein enzyme therapy proposed by John Beard in 1906, this treatment emphasizes the importance of the pancreatic proteolytic enzymes in the body. Like most therapies, this one is significant in helping the human body to heal from the inside.

With the root cause of cancer being lack of oxygen that results in acidity in the human body and cancer cells unable to survive in high levels of oxygen, Dr. Otto Warburg found the solution. This comes into play where antioxidants are involved in killing free radicals, much like using reverse oxidative stress-causing chronic diseases also known as oxygen therapy.

Probiotic foods and supplements also known as the "good bacteria", probiotics are termed as microorganisms that sustain a natural balance in the intestinal microflora of the human body. Introducing these essential herbs into your diet will benefit you greatly.

SIGNIFICANT AMOUNTS of heart friendly, fat-soluble vitamins as well as minerals are still sciences most preferred way to go. They are essential in keeping cancer at a bay. Now, recently, a considerable progress regarding fat-soluble vitamin D3 in preventing cancer has seen tremendous success.

Vitamin C Chelation therapy uses natural compounds or chemicals to detoxify the body. In this case, only holistic doctors and naturopaths embrace the use of chelation therapy since this is not yet approved for most current medicine conditions. In essence, the word "chelate" simply means to grab onto, hence defining the ability of the chelating agents' action on toxins. Usually, this method is used to rid calcium deposits from the arteries. Curcumin has major effects on disease reversal, especially when it comes to cancer. According to a study on cancer cells, curcumin has been proved to have anticancer effects, showing the ability to fight cancer cells and prevent any possible growth of more.

The budwig protocol treatment works pretty simple, by replacing dangerous fats and oils with life-giving saturated fatty acids, thus helping your cells rebuild. According to Dr. Budwig, taking a mixture of cottage cheese flaxseed oil and flax seeds provided the best results. Since cottage is high in sulfur protein, and flax is rich in unsaturated fatty acids. So the body can absorb these essential nutrients faster and easier. Meditation and peace involves eastern techniques like tai chi or feelings of gratitude. Mediation and mental peace as well as a positive outlook can go a long way in life.

Chapter 10
Native American Medicine

Native Americans have known and used numerous plants for medicine over the centuries. Most of the plants and herbs that have been used in the past are still available today, especially in the wild. This means if you know where and what to look, someone can still get the best of these plants by making the most of their herbal medicine beneficial.

Now, the best part is that some of them can also be grown at the backyard, bringing these herbs even closer to home. The dandelion is also referred to as Taraxacum Officinale. It was usually helpful in treating a number of ailments affecting the kidneys, liver, and stomach. The plant further played a significant role as used in the Chinese medicine, with its immunity boosting and antioxidant capabilities. It is best harvested during late spring or early autumn.

Sage also known as Salvia officinalis, the sage was used for diverse medicine and ritualistic purposes. It has seen much use in the kitchen, besides being possibly one of the most commonly grown types. Among its benefits are blood sugar stabilizing effects as well as helping in reducing blood pressure. Moreover, it can be used in treating colds, coughs and digestive issues as well. The upside is that this one is perennial and super easy to grow, especially if planted during spring, right towards the last frost.

Wild cherry is also called Prunus Serotina, and its bark is renowned for possessing anti-inflammatory capabilities. It is also used for treating bronchitis, sore throat, as well as many other respiratory problems. The inner bark is the most useful part of the plant, although quite difficult to harvest if you are not sure on what to do in the process. Most "wild crafting" methods can help in harvesting, and a little research on that could go a long way. This herb can be found in the wild, most possibly between May and June.

Yarrow is also known as Achillea millefolium. The yarrow is popular for its efficiency in blood staunching and efficiency in cleaning as well as healing wounds. Like most other versatile plants in the medicine world, the Yarrow is effective for treating numerous ailments like headaches, hemorrhoids, and even colds when used as tea. The entire plant is useful for its traditional medicine preparations, and the leaves are best harvested during the late spring or early in the summer.

SCIENTIFICALLY KNOWN as the Rosmarinus officinalis, the rosemary has been around for centuries, offering a wide range of benefits. From antioxidants to anti-inflammatory compounds, this plant was essential for treatment of muscle pain, spasms, digestive complications, and hair loss among other purposes. This has also been a major option for promoting healthy brain functioning, as well as posing potential for cancer treatment. Rosemary is easily grown, which adds to its significant medicine and culinary value.

Plants have been used for centuries in the medicine world. These are among the most used herbs and plants in this field.

Chapter 11

Herbs for Better Sex

Everyone wants to have a good time in bed, and face the challenges that come with disruptions. More importantly, you need to ensure you are in a position to make the most of your time with your partner, and this is where these herbs come into play. Take advantage of the benefits they offer and transform your love making for the better.

Sex can't be better than when you have an ideal flow of emotions, intuition, and most importantly, blood flow. This is why this herb is so effective, since it ensures you get the best blood flow, supplying the important sections in your body with the right amount of blood for better functioning.

Now, the best part is that Ginkgo biloba increases your blood circulation without any effect on blood pressure, making it an ideal option for those struggling with erectile dysfunction. The other interesting thing is that biloba works wonders for both men and women alike. The herb is good at stimulating blood circulation to the capillaries under the skin for increased sensitivity.

And like most other herbs out there, biloba is a great solution for your blood flow, but it can cause allergic reactions and digestive upset if you are sensitive to it. In case you are on daily doses of aspirin or anti-clotting drugs, this might not be the right time to take Ginkgo biloba for your safety. The reason for this is that the combination of this herb with drugs can put you at a higher risk of bleeding.

Maca also called the Lepidium meyenii, it is a native plant in Peru. It is essential for increasing stamina, strength, libido, and energy in overall. It can also normalize sex hormones like testosterone, estrogen and progesterone. Maca can also help with fertility problems, irregular menstrual cycles and ease the cycle pain, not to mention regulating menopause transition and suppressing stress.

Ashwagandha also known as Withania somnifera, ashwagandha boosts energy and reduces stress as well as boosting your sperm count. Besides, it is also ideal when it comes to increasing sex hormone production in both males and females alike. Its active principles like anoloid, alkaloids, withanolides and others go a long way in sexual stimulation and offering stamina for increased longevity too.

The only issue here is that you need to take it hours before the action; a few hours prior will work the trick. You also need to mind the fact that it can lead to increased testosterone in the body; this may provoke aggression, especially if you are testosterone sensitive. Your body can also become tolerant to it, making it less effective in the future, so moderation is essential. As such, taking a single 500mg capsule just a few times a week is advisable to start with, as you observe how it works for you.

Chapter 12

Eucalyptus Oils and their Benefits

The eucalyptus has been the source of food for koala beats, but it is also nutrition for wildlife. Perhaps the best part is this plant is also rich in essential oils extracted from its leaves, which poses significant medicinal properties. Also known as the Tasmanian Blue Gum, this tree offers an exceptional advantage, and here are top uses of its oils and their benefits.

A COMBINATION OF THE eucalyptus oil with olive oil or coconut oil can help give your hair a special treat for absolute moisturizing effect. This helps keep dandruff and those itchy scalps at bay. Besides, you can also use it for naturally preventing lice if you don't want to add chemical treatments. According to NYU Medical School, this oil is also efficient in dealing with sinusitis, giving patients faster results.

Whether on your carpet, clothes, or any other fabric in your house, these oils are essential for dealing with the most stubborn spots. Besides, if you have gum on your shoes, you can count on it, but you might need to do a spot test to be sure this won't compromise the quality of the surface.

Eucalyptus is highly helpful in detoxifying your body of microorganisms that can potentially make you sick. By using several drops of its essential oil into the diffuser before you go to sleep, you will benefit from the healing power of this plant in fighting colds easily.

Add several drops into a vacuum or cloth dryer for a little sanitizing and refreshing effect, while still killing mold inside your home. If you wish so, you can always mix the eucalyptus oil with clove and tea oil for air cleansing and mold-free environment in your home.

This oil gives a fresh fragrance to your home, besides adding a touch of crucial anti-microbial properties with every drop. Adding the oil to your laundry detergent, soap, toilet cleaner or mop water could change quite everything.

Treating wounds

With its antiseptic and antimicrobial properties, this oil is effective in treating burns, wounds, abrasions, sores, cuts, scrapes among others. What's more, you can also use it on bug bites. Use it along with a (natural) pain reliever in the affected area, and it will help keep it free of infection and aid in faster healing. From dog beds to smelly shoes and virtually any other odor around, you can fix things easier with the use of these oils in washing your items. Soak a rag in eucalyptus oil and water, then dry it in the sun and use it for washing. Alternatively, you can go for lemon oil or tea tree to beat the stench.

Such respiratory problems like bronchitis, asthma and pneumonia among others can prove difficult to deal with. But eucalyptus oil comes in handy dilating blood vessels like in the case of asthma. Just mix it with coconut oil, peppermint oil and apply on the upper side of your chest.

Chapter 13

Remedies for Allergies

Most people are allergic to one thing or the other, sometimes it may seem as a way of life, but when the situation is critical, things are never that easy. Going for a scientific remedy can be reliable as well as a natural way.

If there is one old remedy for several health conditions out there, it has to be apple cider vinegar. It helps with allergy and heartburn quite well. The secret behind this remedy is its ability to suppress production of mucus and cleaning the lymph system. Besides, it can be a great relief if you have weight loss or digestion problems to deal with, this will come to your rescue.

Quercetin natural bioflavonoid allegedly helps in stabilizing mast cells, hence preventing release of histamine. Besides, the herb is highly antioxidant that helps reduce inflammation and can be a long-term solution if taken about four to six weeks before allergy season to avert the symptoms.

THE NETTLE LEAF IS a great natural antihistamine for naturally blocking production of histamine in the body. The herb can grow in several places, and you can make it into a tea or a tincture. However, if you are looking for allergy relief, capsules made from this herb may be the best way to go, and mostly the most efficient option at your disposal. A transition in your diet may come as a last result, but not the least of course. GAPS diet has been observed to reduce allergic symptoms, especially severe food allergies in children.

Usually, allergies result from issues of imbalance especially within the immunity system, causing the body to react excessively towards stimuli. According to research, bacteria in the gut can contribute to lower cases of allergies. As such, taking measures to balance the bacteria in the gut and consumption of beneficial bacteria can aid in solving this problem. Local honey is not backed by scientific research as such, but the hands-on experiments done by people have proved promising. The theory behind it is that consumption of honey from your locality could enable the body adapt to the environmental allergens that you are exposed to. Working as more of a natural allergy vaccine, this does not seem to have side effects.

Fighting allergy symptoms may never be that easy, but you can always be smart enough if you know where to turn, also be sure to get tested for allergens by your physician.

Chapter 14
Herbs to Unclog Your Arteries

Having poor blood circulation is the last thing any physician will take easy. This can be a crisis if it is not well handled from the very onset. Luckily, you can always take charge and make things work for you, thanks to herbs that you can count on. But before getting into details, let's look at the symptoms of poor blood circulation first.

- Cold hands and fingers
- Frequent headaches
- Extreme numbness in some parts of the body
- Regular dizziness
- Cold feet and toes
- Lack of energy
- Water retention on feet
- Memory loss, etc.

GINKGO BILOBA, EXTRACTED from one of the most ancient trees around, this potent antioxidant, initially used to improve memory loss and treat other blood disorders. Green tea has a powerful medicinal value in improving the cells responsible for lining the capillaries. Besides, it can also help reduce the risk of heart disease or cancer, as well as reducing the risk of coronary artery and stroke. This is also great for improving your blood flow.

Parsley herb can be found in several supplements, thanks to its capability to be used as a natural vasodilator, opening up blood pathways throughout the body and its high level of vitamin C and B12 enhancing this important process.

Bilberry is usually used for treating diarrhea, it can also help improve any cases of blood coruscation with its potent for blood thinning. It is useful for patients with chronic venous insufficiency in case the veins around the legs become damaged and unable to carry blood to the heart as intended.

Cayenne pepper has been used in medicine for centuries, thanks to a chemical known as capsaicin, which gives the herb its outstanding heat.

Willow bark, a salicin contained in this herb is similar to aspirin, and has been used in the medicine world since 40 B.C, treating inflammation and pain. This herb helps thin the blood for better circulation, although the herb is still subject to more research and safety. Hawthorn can be found in most supplements. It helps with the circulatory system with the regulation of the heart rate as well as enhancing blood flow from the heart. Horse chestnut can be catastrophic if eaten raw, it is useful for treating circulation problems if well processed.

Ginger is responsible for opening up blood vessels to allow more blood passing through, which earns it the name vasodilator. And since the herb is also anti-viral and packed with anti-inflammatory properties, it can double as a remedy for flu and cold or joint problems. Besides, a cup of ginger tea a day could help boost your immune system as well. So you can go out there, grab your favorite herb, and regain charge of your blood circulation as well as getting rid of other problems along the way.

Chapter 15

Native American Natural Herbs

MEDICINE MEN IN NATIVE America used means more similar to Asian medicine, using herbal remedies as well as other cutting-edge treatment options. The conventional holistic approach was largely depended on the use of plants, harnessing their outstanding benefits. The list of herbs, flowers, fruits and trees used is quite a long one, but here are the top ten methods that were usually used.

Alfalfa relieves digestion and boosts blood clotting. It was usually employed in treating bladder and kidney conditions, arthritis as well as bone strength and enhancing the immunity system. Blackberry when crushed, the roots, leaves and bark of this plant was useful in treating diarrhea, stimulating metabolism and reducing inflammation. When used as a gargle, it was helpful in treating mouth ulcers, sore throat, and gum inflammation.

Aspen, the xylem of this plant was widely used for treating fever, pain and coughs. Besides, its salicin content is useful as a foundation ingredient used in aspirin. An essential natural remedy for fever and headaches for example severe migraines, it is also effective in solving digestion problems, asthma and muscle as well as joint pains among other uses.

Beeswax was useful in treating insect bites like bee stings, and treatment for burns. It was only used externally. Black raspberry plant's roots were crushed for use as chewed, boiled or tea. It helped relieve diarrhea, coughs, and treat normal distress in the intestines.

Echinacea/ coneflower medicine was largely used in strengthening the immune system, as well as fighting infections and fever. Besides, it doubles as an antiseptic and a treatment for coughs, flu and colds. Aloe thick leaves of this cactus-like plant were squeezed to provide thick sap for treating burns, wounds and insect bites.

Eucalyptus plant's roots and leaves produce oil that was used for common treatment purposes, especially after it was infused in tea. It could treat sore throat, coughs, flu and fever.

Buckwheat seeds were essential in lowering blood pressure, enhancing blood clotting and relieving diarrhea. It was used in soup or as porridge. Chokecherry usually considered an all-in-one treatment. Native Americans would put, dry, and crush the berries, then use them as a variety of ailments. This helped in treating nausea, coughs, flu, colds, diarrhea, and inflammation to mention but a few. However, care is essential as the pit of these cherry can be poisonous if highly concentrated.

Bee pollen can be mixed with food to provide a boost in the energy and the immunity system, as well as aiding in digestion. But for those who are allergic to bee stings, this one can cause allergic reaction as well. Cayenne used as pods helped in relieving pain, digestive distress and treating arthritis as well. Their powder was also applied in wounds to increase blood flow and provide antiseptic effects, as well as numbing the pain. Chamomile used as tea, this herb's flowers and leaves were essential in treating intestinal problems and nausea.

Fennel plant has a licorice flavor, and is essential for treating sore throat, coughs and aiding in digestion. It can be chewed or used in tea. Other remedies include relief for diarrhea, and general use for treating colds, a relief for headaches and eyes. The list of conventional Native American natural herbs is almost endless, extending to over thirty of the options used back then. Most of them are useful even today, like ginseng, ginger root and feverwort, you can hardly exhaust the alternatives.

Chapter 16
Detoxifying Herbs

Detoxification is one of the most important things you can do for your body. Some of these herbs have been used for years for several ailments, and in different cultures. The best part is these herbs have held on through time, and are still in used in most of the body cleansing products on the market.

Dandelion has been used for centuries, with virtually all its parts used for various ailments. From enhancing bowel regularity to promoting reliable dehydration levels, joint discomfort, and used as a tea as well. Besides, the herb comes in handy with the body immunity system and detoxification, while the root is useful for liver cleansing.

Gum extracted from the bark of an acacia plant has been useful for improving electrolyte absorption, adding bulk to the movements in the bowel, thus relieving diarrhea symptoms. The herb is also essential for use as a hydrocolloid. This is used as an emulsifier for stabilizing and facilitating synergy between ingredients that are difficult to mix.

Organic milk thistle helps the gall bladder as well as the liver in bile production for improved digestion process. The herb is essential ingredient in Livatrex, a popular cleansing product for the liver and gallbladder.

Wormwood, this herb has seen its fair share of difficulties in the medicine world; it is still going strong, being used as a remedy for pinworms and roundworms. Moreover, it is renowned for its historical use as a digestion aid.

Black walnut is packed with three active agents, tannins, juglone and iodine. These make it a go to choice when it comes to natural health practices, with the juglone more potent with natural defense capabilities. Iodine is significant for almost all life forms, with an unsurpassed help in reducing most harmful organisms' lifespan. The tannins are crucial for keeping these organisms at bay altogether.

Alfalfa herb leaves have been used for years, treating several infections. To others, this was an aid to the body in fighting stomach ulcers not to mention its use for appetite stimulation.

Talk of helping removal of toxic metals accumulating in the body's organ tissue. Cilantro is also known for its natural cleansing agents with compounds for binding toxic materials and helping pull them from different tissues.

Eucalyptus is popular for its cleansing abilities, especially for the lungs. Its expectorant properties help fight viral and bacterial attacks and can be useful for chest congestion or a remedy for a stuffy nose. The calming and soothing properties give this herb its unique edge.

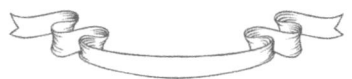

PEPPERMINT SOOTHING quality is essential for treating coughs, colds and flu. It can also help in cases of sinus irritation or sore throat, and helps the body fight harmful organisms. In addition, if you are looking for a lung cleansing solution, this might well be the one for you.

Stinging Nettle is popular for its repulsion to organisms, as well as being resistant to swelling and systematic redness. It is also rich in antioxidants and can help in promoting normal blood pressure.

Chapter 17
Sage in Herbal Medicine

S age is one of the herbs that have been around the longest. It has been vastly used in the culinary and medical fields. The Egyptians used it for fertility, and a Greeks physician stated the effects of Sage in stopping bleeding in wounds and cleaning ulcers as well as treating sores. The physician, Dioscorides, further recommends the use of this herb's juice in warm water, useful for treating coughs and hoarseness. Generally, sage has seen much action in the medication world, and here are some of the qualities that have given the herb much recognition.

Besides being used in other countries, Sage is regarded in Germany for treating inflammations, by being applied as a rinse or gargled. The herbs tincture, essential oils as well as extract are important for preparation of medicine for mouth, gastrointestinal remedies (used in fluid), and throat. The herbs anti-inflammatory properties are attributed to the herb's rosmarinic acid. In Germany, this herb has been used as internal dosage for sweating and gastrointestinal upsets, and externally on throat and mouth.

From dental abscesses, throat infections, infected gums, to mouth ulcers, Sage has been effective in a diversity of conditions. Sage contains phenolic acids, which are potentially effective for use against serious staphylococcus aureus. This has seen the herb's oil used against Escherichia coli as well as Salmonella species. Sage has also been effective in treating yeasts and filamentous fungi like Candida albicans. Besides, the herb has an outstanding astringent action resulting from its tannin rich nature, which means it can be essential for treating infantile diarrhea. For the antiseptic effect, sage helps in treating intestinal infection.

Among the wide number of conditions that sage can help with is the condition of menopause symptoms like night sweats, hot flashes, and other estrogenic effects.

From reducing griping and different symptoms of indigestion, sage can help with multiple conditions when taken as a carminative. Besides, the herb can also be used in treating dysmenorrhea, and a bitter component in this herb is essential for stimulating secretions in upper digestive sections, as well as bile flow, intestinal mobility and pancreatic function. On the other end, its volatile oil possesses a stimulating and carminative effect on the digestive system.

Among the wide range of conditions that sage can be used on is the general relaxant effect of the herb. This means that sage can be used for treating nervousness, excitability and dizziness among other.

Sage has proved to be effective for a number of conditions, and muscle tension is no exception. This herb possesses an antispasmodic action, and this has been proven to reduce tension in the muscles. It further is used on counter asthma attack in a steam inhalation. Besides, it helps remove mucus congestion in the airways, helping prevent or monitor secondary infections.

Just like rosemary, sage is essential in improving functioning of the brain as well as memory retention. According to a study conducted on twenty volunteers, sage oil showed improvement in the ability to recall words and increasing attention speed. Besides, sage's constituents have been on the line of investigation in search for new drugs that can be used in treating Alzheimer's disease, and has shown potential effects.

Much has been achieved with sage, and it is apparently potential for even more opportunities in the future. When it comes to this herb's significance, there is much significance in the quest for herbal medicine.

Chapter 18

Hydroponic Herb Garden

Q uite often, you feel the urge to grow veggies and maybe herbs at your backyard, but have you ever figured out putting up a hydroponic garden? Hydroponic is ideal for production of medicinal and culinary herbs. Perhaps the best part about these gardens is that herbs not only grow faster, but also have more aroma than the ones grown in a conventional garden. According to research, the herbs can be 20 to 40% more aromatic over the ones grown in the field. And if you want a consistent high quality produce from a small space, this is the way to go.

IF YOU ARE AIMING TO use this method at home, then a small Ebb and flow system is the ideal option. Here, the plants will be held in a flood table, inside plastic pots, and then the reservoirs will be positioned beneath. A submersible pump can be run on a timer to get rid of the waste gases as well as supplying the roots with water rich in nutrients. Once the timer is off, water will withdraw back to the reservoir, and pull fresh oxygen to the herbs' roots. You can do this after every fifteen minutes, three or four times in a day.

With the herbs almost primarily vegetative, using grow formula nutrient rich in high nitrogen and relatively lower phosphorus is always an excellent ratio to work with for most of these herbs. Usually, a low-to-medium measure of electrical conductivity for measuring the strength of nutrients can be handy. Any measure from 1.2 to 1.8 with a bit of acidic PH at around 5.8 to 6.4 is a great deal when growing culinary herbs. If you want to keep the measurements of these aspects, you can always go for PH pens and EC meters, which won't eat into your budget.

When growing herbs indoors, most of them require full spectrum light with an abundance of blue towards the end. You can go for T-5 high output fluorescent or metal halide lights, they always work wonders in this settings. If you can get a new 315 watt ceramic type metal halide or a 400 watt HID light system (HPS), you can be able to cover up to 4 x 4 foot square area. If you are going to use a 1000 watt HID light system, you will have 6X6 feet square covered. It is advisable to keep the lighting system about one foot to a foot and a half over the tips of the herbs, and then raise the lights with the growth of the plants. Especially for the fluorescent lamps with high output like the T-5, you can place them closer to the plants as they run cooler.

An oscillating fan can also help in your herb garden, as ideal air movement will ensure the plants are cool and have sufficient supply of carbon dioxide, which helps in photosynthesis. Keeping the temperature at about 70 to 75 degrees and a relative humidity of about 40 to 60% can be a great idea.

Plants can be tough enough to withstand difficult conditions sometime, especially when it comes to the environmental conditions and fertilization. It is believed that too much attention to detail into these aspects might weaken the plants. So you can give them a little stress to ensure they harden, but care is necessary though.

Chapter 19

Boost Your Immunity and Fight Infection with Antiviral herbs

Viruses are infectious microorganisms that replicate within the cells of an organism, and are capable of attacking virtually all life forms, single celled and multicellular alike. What's more, they exist in various ecosystems, and can transfer genetic material and reproduce through natural selection. However, these organisms do not have a definite cell structure. These organisms can spread in several ways, either through blood sucking insects in animals, others through sneezing and coughing, or spread by fecal-oral means.

The worst part is that antibiotics may not be of much help, and vaccines are unreliable as some viruses can be evasive. But fortunately, antiviral herbs are essential in suppressing the microorganisms' development, not to mention that herbs pose fewer chances for side effects. Besides, most of these herbs can boost your immune system too, helping the body keep viral pathogens at bay. This is where herbs outweigh the antiviral drugs, as they don't target a specific group of pathogens. This helps to prevent the evasive mutation of viruses that help the organisms become difficult to treat. Well, here are top ten antiviral herbs for dealing with a virus.

Echinacea is an all-time herb for its immune support and general health benefits. Phytochemicals in this herb are potent of reducing virus tumors and infections, with a compound Echinacea in this herb inhibiting virus and bacteria from entering healthy cells and significantly reducing any chances of infections.

Elderberry is a long renowned herb for its popularity among many cultures, thanks to its benefits in medicine. The herb can help fight herpes, influenza, and bacterial as well as viral infections.

Garlic, and some compounds found in the herb has been proven highly effective in killing numerous microorganisms that cause rare and common infections alike. Garlic is known for healing problems like pneumonia, tuberculosis, herpes and thrush. Besides, thanks to the antiviral properties, this herb is effective in treating eye infection as well as a natural remedy against ear infection.

Calendula flower petals have been essential for medicinal use from the 12th century. The herb is high in flavonoids, plant-based antioxidants for protecting cells from damage by radicals. Used when dry, the petals of this herb are also essential for fighting bacteria, viruses and inflammation. They also help on burns, infections, healing cuts, and wounds.

Cat's claw roots and bark have been used in South America for years in treating problems like stomach ulcers, fevers, digestive complications and dysentery. The herb is also a remedy for arthritis and ulcers symptoms, as well as herpes.

Astragalus has been used in traditional Chinese medicine as an antiviral herb for hundreds of years. The herb was also mainly used for boosting the body's immunity system, something that scientists have also approved, and suggest that the herb can also be used for cold and flu prevention.

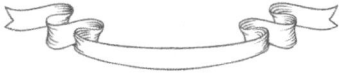

GINGER'S ABILITY TO enhance the body's immune system has been recognized since time immemorial. The herb's ability to heat the body helps prevent accumulation of toxins in the organs. Ginger is also known to cleanse the lymph system and the body's sewage system.

Olive leaf is potent with antiviral properties; this herb is able of treating the common cold as well as other serious viruses like Candida symptoms, pneumonia, meningitis, gonorrhea, hepatitis B and tuberculosis. Moreover, it is essential for treating urinary tract infections, ear, dental and shingles.

Licorice has also been the go-to option for treatment of HIV, hepatitis C, and influenza.

Oregano oil is rich in carvacrol and thymol compounds, potent with antifungal and antibacterial properties. Carvacrol helps with viral infections, allergies, tumors and disease causing inflammation.

Chapter 20

Herbal and Supplement Treatments for Diabetes

Treating diabetes can be a tricky affair, especially if you do not have the right medication handy. The good news is, there are a lot of herbs and supplements that you can turn to and get the problem reduced.

BILBERRY IS KNOWN FOR protecting nerves and eyes, and a dosage of 80 to 1230 milligrams of its extract a day is recommended. The herb contains potent antioxidants known as anthocyanins in both the fruits and leaves. This prevents damage to minute blood vessels, which could lead to retinopathy and nerve pain. Besides, according to study conducted on animals, Bilberry can also lower blood sugar.

Bitter melon is used for lowering blood, and usually a 50 to 100 milliliter of the juice goes for a daily dosage. The juice is believed to enhance the use of glucose in cells as well as blocking absorption of sugar in the intestines. Philippine researchers noted that someone taking bitter melon capsules could achieve lower blood sugar than another one taking placebo. Though slight, the change can be consistent.

Magnesium is also used for lowering blood sugar, with a dosage of 250 to 350 milligrams a day recommended. Deficiency of this mineral is popular among diabetic people. It could mean high blood sugar levels and resistance to insulin. According to some studies, a magnesium supplement can improve the functioning of insulin as well as reducing blood levels, but it is advisable to check with your doctor before using this supplement.

Prickly pear cactus is another blood sugar lowering supplement with a required daily dose of half a cup of cooked cactus fruit. The ripe fruit is known to lower blood sugar levels, thanks to some components that are believed to work similarly as insulin. It can be found on grocery stores or as juice or powder at most heath stores. It is also rich in fiber, making it a great choice for diabetic patients' diet.

YOU SHOULD CONSULT your doctor before you consider adding any medication to your collection, especially in cases where the dose might lower your blood sugar. It is also advisable you keep checking your blood sugar often and work with your physician in adjusting your dosage. If there is no change in a month or two, you can stop using money on the medicine.

The main use of Gamma-linolenic acid is easing nerve pain, and a daily dose of 270 to 540 milligrams is recommended. Also known as GLA, this is a fatty acid from evening primrose oil. It is believed that diabetic people have lower GLA, and studies suggest that the supplement can go a long way in either reducing or preventing nerve pain that comes with the disease.

Alpha-lipoic acid is useful for lowering blood sugar and easing nerve pain. Also known as ALA, the substance neutralizes several radical types in the body. These could result from high blood sugar, and can cause damage to the nerves alongside other complications. The substance is also capable of helping muscle cells in helping with blood sugar levels.

GINSENG ALSO HELPS in reducing blood sugar, and requires a dosage of 1 to 3 grams daily, either in tablet or capsule form. It can also be taken as tincture, with 3 to 5 milligrams required for every day dose. Ginseng is known for boosting immunity and fighting diseases. It has been found to slow carbohydrates absorption, which in turn increases the ability of the cells to utilize glucose; while on the other hand, it enhances the secretion of insulin from the pancreas.

FENUGREEK IS KNOWN for lowering blood sugar, and one is required to take a dose of 5 to 30 grams with every meal. Alternatively, it can be taken in quantities of 15 to 90 grams with each meal in a day. Fenugreek seeds are used in Indian cooking, and are known to lower blood sugar, reducing cholesterol levels as well as increasing sensitivity in insulin. The effects are partly related to the seeds' high fiber content. Besides, they are also rich in amino acids, presumed to enhance insulin release in the body.

Chromium is also known for its blood sugar reducing ability, if taken in daily doses of 200 micrograms. The trace mineral boosts insulin action and takes part in metabolism of fat, carbohydrates and proteins. According to studies, it is ideal for optimizing blood sugar, but its effects are only limited to people with its deficit.

Remember, it is always wise advisable that you check with your physician before switching to any medication.

Chapter 21

Herbal Remedies for Bedwetting

Bedwetting makes the victim embarrassed. Bedwetting is also known as enuresis. In children, bedwetting occurs as a result of an immature bladder. The bladder size is too small to hold high quantities of urine.

It is important to handle anyone with bedwetting problems carefully. Love and care should be shown during periods of discussion about the topic. This encourages children that the situation will pass. It is usually temporary.

Why Bedwetting Happens in Teens and Adults

Bedwetting also affects some teens and adults. The known reasons for bedwetting among adults is

- Diseases, e.g., UTIs and diabetes
- Deep sleep
- Low levels of ADH (an antidiuretic hormone)
- Small-sized bladder
- Emotional distress in teens or stress

Many bedwetting reduction techniques are used. They usually attempt at reducing the fluid amount produced in order not to strain the bladder. Bladder training is also used.

Fortunately, these simple herbs do not require complicated regimes or complex skills.

Effective Herbs against Bedwetting

These herbal options serve to aid bedwetting.

1. Cinnamon
2. Fennel seeds

3. Olive leaf
4. Corn silk
5. Saw Palmetto
6. Horsetail, oak bark, and bearberry herbal tea
7. Gooseberries
8. Cranberry Juice

Cinnamon

Children are given a cinnamon stick to chew. Cinnamon is effective against bed wetting. Alternatively, cinnamon powder can be sprinkled on toast. Fennel seeds are used as a spice. They can be used to make an herbal tea or placed in food. They are effective against bedwetting in adults. Olive leaf has antimicrobial properties. The olive leaf is used to treat bladder infections. Some infections exacerbate bedwetting. Treating the underlying problem usually solves bedwetting complications. Corn silk is the name given to that part of corn that looks like shiny fibers protruding from the corn ear.

Corn silk tea is a nutrition rich (full of potassium), and it has a sweet flavor which is mild. It is used to treat incontinence and UTIs. It is an anti-inflammatory agent in treating UTI infections. Corn silk also regulates blood sugar. It helps in the production of insulin in the body. The tea is effective in lowering the blood sugar levels thus controlling diabetes. Diabetes can cause bedwetting. After corn silk manages the sugar levels, bedwetting stops completely.

Saw palmetto extract has been used by several different traditional medicine cultures to treat urogenital infections. It is prescribed for bedwetting since it is associated with the reproductive system. It is useful in treating bedwetting in adult males. Saw Palmetto can be found as supplements sold in major stores.

Horsetail, Oak bark, and Bearberry Herbal Tea

This is an ancient Ayurvedic practice of combining three herbs in moderate quantities to make an herbal tea. It has proven to be effective against stopping urine flow at night. Indian gooseberries are also called

Amla. They are green in color. Taking Indian gooseberries has also been a proven Ayurvedic practice against bedwetting. Cranberry juice is also an efficient and tasty method against bedwetting.

Chapter 22
Asthma

A sthmatics will tell you that asthma brings along hefty bills in pharmaceutical drugs aimed at reducing the symptoms. However, these drugs usually end up creating recurring bills since they do not cure asthma. There is no known cure for asthma. The drugs only manage symptoms. Natural remedies have almost no harmful side effects unless if these natural herbs are used by individuals with other ailments that react negatively to the herbs. Natural does not necessarily mean safe. Information about herbs is necessary.

Asthma Triggers and Symptoms

The exact cause of asthma is unknown. Only the factors that trigger reactions have been identified. Triggers include:

- Air pollution
- Allergens
- Emotional conditions
- Weather conditions
- Respiratory infections

However, natural remedies are cost effective and provide the highly needed relief from severe asthma symptoms. Some herbs that have been used to manage asthma include: Ginkgo Biloba has anti-inflammatory properties, and it is an antihistamine in nature. Since one symptom of asthma is inflammation and sensitivity of the airway to pollen and air contaminants, Ginkgo Biloba is essential for the management of inflammation and allergic reactions.

Ginkgo Biloba inhibits platelet Activating Factor (PAF).PAF is a mediator in any reactions to stimuli by inflammatory cells, which increase in size. PAF interferes with the inflammation process, thus controlling, e.g., the blocking of airways that cause difficulty in breathing and shortness of breath. The symptom is relieved because Ginkgo inhibits it due to the PAF property.

Slippery elm is an herb that thins phlegm. Since phlegm clogs the air passage in Asthma, slippery elm manages the mucus and reduces wheezing in Asthma patients. It also controls coughing and loosens chest muscles.

Ginger also has anti-inflammatory properties that act on the smooth muscle. Ginger works by reducing muscle constriction, which causes asthmatic attacks. The patient encounters significant resistance when breathing. Ginger relaxes the constricted muscles hence, allowing adequate passage of air in and out of the lung alveoli.

Turmeric is also a root that belongs to the same family as ginger. It is also a spice, and has medicinal values. Medically, it has diarylheptanoids as the active ingredients. One diarylheptanoid chemical is Curcumin. Curcumin is an anti-inflammatory agent. This property works on the inflammation induced in air passages in Asthmatic attacks and helps to reverse inflammation. This herb allows easier breathing thus loosening the muscles that make someone feel tightness in the chest area.

Garlic is also an herb with anti-inflammatory properties. It has been used over a period of many years to manage cardiovascular anomalies. Garlic efficacy in managing the symptoms of asthma is currently in study. There is no concrete evidence. However, its anti-inflammatory properties are effective in controlling asthmatic attacks.

In Traditional Chinese Medicine, garlic is used because it also possesses antibiotic and antiviral properties, which keep respiratory infections at bay. It is also believed to boost immunity. It controls wheezing by clearing the lung congestion.

Chapter 23
The Lobelia Herb

Lobelia is known as Indian tobacco. Its scientific name is Lobelia inflata. It is also known as the puke weed in layman language. It is an herb found in Eastern North America. It is known as the puke weed because doctors induce vomiting in their patients so that any toxin in the gut could be eliminated. This was common in the 19th Century.

Lobelia is an annual or a biennial plant that grows to about 50-100cm. It has ovate leaves, which are about 8 cm long. Its flowers are violet with a yellow tint on the inside. Its stem is hairy, and the leaves are toothed. This herb is commonly used in homeopathy, a home treatment routine that is an alternative medicine option. It is employed in small doses since large prescription amounts may cause adverse effects such as rapid heartbeat, mental confusion, convulsions, coma, and death.

Small doses are prescribed to clear the airway of mucus. The other side effects of Lobelia include diarrhea, sweating, vomiting, nausea, and tremors. There are no adequate scientific studies to back up claims of the mentioned medicinal attributes of Lobelia. However, since there is evidence of historical success, some herbalists include Lobelia as part of the treatment for Asthma. The Cherokee (Native Americans) used to burn the leaves of the Lobelia plant to get rid of gnats.

It was once thought that Lobelia plant contained Lobeline as an active ingredient. Hence, Lobeline was used as a substitute for nicotine in products aimed at alleviating nicotine addiction. It soon became evident that products with Lobeline were not effective in curbing nicotine dependence. Since people were not getting any help in quitting smoking, the FDA (US) banned products with Lobeline in 1993.

Scientists now believe that Lobeline affects the release of a chemical in the brain called Dopamine. Dopamine is responsible for causing drug addiction in patients. Researchers suggest that Lobeline may reduce nicotine addiction if it affects Dopamine release. However, there are no studies to support these claims.

It is suggested that Asthma, Bronchitis, and Coughs can be treated using a combination of the Lobelia herb and other herbs.

In homeopathic medicine, Lobelia is prescribed for quitting smoking, insect bites, ringworm infection, poison ivy rash, bruises, vomiting, muscle relaxation, nausea and other respiratory infections. Lobelia is available as an herbal tea, tinctures, capsules and liquid extract. It can also be applied topically as an ointment or a lotion.

Some herbs require the supervision of a medical practitioner. Not all herbs are safe to use in moderate or large quantities. Moderation expertise is needed in these cases. Lobelia is an herb that needs such care since it is a potentially toxic herb and massive amounts ingested, can lead to death. Lobelia is known to irritate the gastrointestinal tract. It may, therefore, worsen the symptoms of ulcers and other diseases associated with the GI tract such as the bowel Inflammatory Disease.

People with heart infections and anomalies, high blood pressure, kidney and liver complications, paralysis, shortness of breath, seizures, sensitivity to tobacco and anyone in shock recovery at any stage should not use Lobelia in any form, even in tea. Expectant mothers and breastfeeding women are also advised against using any form of Lobelia.

Chapter 24

Herpes Simplex 2

A lot of research has been carried out on both the HSV-1 and HSV-2 virus. HSV-1 is an oral disease that causes breakouts in cold sores. HSV-2 is genital herpes. HSV-1 is transmitted through body fluids in toothbrushes, towels, and acts of kissing. HSV-2 is transmitted via skin to skin contact. It is sexually transmitted.

It's hard to target the HSV virus using medication since it hides in the neurons located at the spinal base. The body does not attack these neurons, even when affected because they are hard to regenerate. There is no cure for the HSV virus, but the symptoms are managed by available treatments. Herbal medication reduces the frequency of HSV-2 outbreaks. Once infected, HSV stays in the body. It stays for life. The outbreaks are the menace; otherwise, it is a dormant virus.

Outbreak Triggers

• Triggers of HSV outbreaks include:

• Stress

• Compromised immunity resulting from infections

HSV-2 Symptoms

These associated symptoms usually occur during outbreaks.

Symptoms of Herpes Simplex 2 (HSV-2) include:

Sores around the genitalia

Flu-like symptoms

Painful or not sores may exhibit

Pain when passing urine

Irritation and itching around the genitalia

Herbs that are documented as effective against HSV-2 outbreaks include: Olive leaf has demonstrated anti-viral properties. It prevents how HSV virus replicates in the body. Olive leaf also can enter infected cells and change their DNA and RNA material. Olive leaf also boosts the immune system and fights fungal and yeast infections.

Echinacea herb works in conjunction of another herb called Andrographis to strengthen the immune system and target virally infected cells. The herbal combination also provides relief to the affected mucous membranes by sores. The Andrographis herb is a potent immune enhancer. HSV-2 outbreaks commonly occur in an immunocompromised environment. It is important to keep the immune system strengthened to avoid outbreaks.

Andrographis interferes with viral replication and it also prevents healthy cells from being infected. It inhibits the spread of infection. Lemon Balm may also be known as Bee balm, Balm mint. Balm mint is applied on the site of sores outbreak before the sores erupt. It is effective in killing 97.2% of the virus. Peppermint possesses strong anti-viral properties which act against HSV-2. It stops the virus from replication.

Prunella is a potent antiviral herb. It can be used as a tea before an outbreak as a preventative measure. Sage is also a strong antiviral herb. It can be used as a tea before an outbreak as a preventative measure.

Rosemary has antiviral properties that attack the HSV-2 virus. It can be used as a tea before an outbreak as a preventative measure. Thyme is an antiviral botanical which attacks the HSV-2 virus. It can be used as a tea before an outbreak as a preventative measure.

Rhubarb Root is a topical cream from a rhubarb root is effective in treating sores. When the sage herb is combined with rhubarb to make a topical cream, it is effective. Sage alone is ineffective. A tincture from the rhubarb root works better than acyclovir, a medicine used in hospitals to treat HSV-2.

Siberian ginseng reduces the duration of an outbreak, its severity and frequency of outbreaks. Siberian ginseng interacts with several medications. A doctor should be consulted before using Siberian ginseng. It should not be mixed with blood thinner medication. People with high blood pressure, hormone-related cancers, sleep apnea, narcolepsy mania, pregnant or breastfeeding mothers should not use Siberian ginseng.

Aloe gel works efficiently in the healing process of genital sores. Preliminary evidence points out faster healing time in genital lesions in men.

Many marine plants contain active chemicals essential for metabolism that exhibit anti-HSV activity. More research is underway. The biodiversity can be utilized in HSV management as supplements. Natural remedies for HSV-2 symptoms have been backed by scientific research.

Chapter 25

Herbs to Use in Steam Baths

S team baths utilize aromatherapy. Aromatherapy is involves inhaling the scents produced by essential oils or dried herbs that are infused in steam baths. Steam baths also promote sweating which cleanses the body of toxins. Steam baths relax the body system for later optimum functionality. Steam baths also help in soothing chest infections and decongesting a blocked respiratory system.

Steam baths are good in overcoming any symptoms of acne, treating dry and chapped skin, reducing skin irritations, treating eczema, relieving muscular pain and tension; steam also helps in reducing phlegm buildup, managing coughs, managing bronchitis and Asthma breathing difficulties.

Essential Oils and Herbs used in steam Baths

Some common herbs used in steam baths include:

1. Eucalyptus
2. Lemon oil
3. Pine
4. Chamomile
5. Sage
6. Lavender
7. Juniper
8. Peppermint/Mint
9. Birch
10. Sandalwood
11. Tea Tree oils
12. Evening primrose oil

- Eucalyptus

This herb is useful for opening up the chest Airways. It helps to alleviate the symptoms of common colds, sore throats, and coughs.

- Lemon Oil

The antidepressants in this oil ensure good moods and a relaxed mental state is achieved after a steam bath. Lemon oil is also a tonic and anti-inflammatory oil. Lemon herb is also an excellent detoxifier and body cleanser.

- Pine

The smell of natural forests is relaxing, and pine oil achieves this state. An individual feels refreshed and calm. Pine scent is perfect for combating respiratory infections and for promoting better breathing.

- Chamomile

This essential oil or dried herb is useful for the treatment of any skin infections. It is also a remedy for sunburns.

- Sage

Sage acts as a deodorant. It gets rid of body odor. It reduces excessive perspiration. Sage is useful for the treatment of inflammation. Sage has antioxidant properties. Hence it prevents aging effects on the skin. Consistent steam baths infused with sage is cosmetic.

- Lavender

Lavender aids sleeping. It has sedative properties. Lavender is applied on bruises, and it is also used to clean cuts. It also soothes skin irritations. It promotes healing for skin issues when infused in steam baths.

- Juniper

Juniper oils have diuretic properties. Juniper encourages the expulsion of urine from the body. Salt and excessive water are eliminated from the body through the removal of increased urine.

- Peppermint

If you need nausea relief, try peppermint infused steam baths. Peppermint also cures headaches, soothes stomach aches and reduces fevers. Peppermint herbs calm the nervous system and reduce physical aches. The calming effects mild emotional responses.

Peppermint has anti- inflammatory properties that reduce arthritic pain.

- Birch

This herb is known to reduce bouts of depression, disinfect and relieve pain. It also has calming effects.

- Sandalwood

For that calm after a stress filled day, use sandalwood oil.

- Tea Tree Oils

This oil treats skin conditions. It has antiseptic properties.

- Evening Primrose oil

Another great anti-aging natural herb is evening primrose. Its oil is excellent for ingestion and topical application such as for use in steam baths. It helps to firm skin, reduce skin roughness and make skin resistant to the strain effects of fatigue.

Chapter 26

Herbal Remedies for Natural Pain Relief

Pain can ruin your day. Instead of depending on the many over-the-counter (OTC) pain medications easily available in drug stores, go herbal. While OTC drugs have been linked to addiction and deaths in the past, herbal pain relievers have not caused any addiction or deaths. Herbal medication has side effects and may interact with other medication, but with information on how to use herbs to get to healthy, you should be safe.

One side effect of herbal medication such as willow bark is its ability to thin blood. If ingested with a blood thinning medication, it can result in excessive bleeding, if an injury occurs. White Willow Bark has been used to reduce inflammation and fever. It also reduces lower back pain. It has the active ingredient as salicin which is used in most pain- relief medications for inflammation and back pain.

The white willow bark can be utilized as a tea, as capsules, or tinctures. The white willow bark can be brewed as a tea to relieve headaches.

The white willow bark is also used to calm osteoarthritis pain and lower back pain. Its side effects include blood thinning, stomach upsets or slowing down the kidneys. Ginger is a natural anti-inflammatory agent. It has been hailed as effective against muscle and joint pain, related muscle soreness, nausea, menstrual cramps, and headaches. Ginger can be taken as a tea. Ginger also helps with proper blood circulation. Ginger compresses have also been documented as effective against pain.

Capsaicin is the active ingredient against pain in red hot chili peppers. It takes time for sufficient results to be realized. It is not advisable to eat chilies for any fast relief of pain. Capsaicin alleviates pain by interfering with the secretion of a substance that transmits pain sensations to the CNS. Valerian root has been used as an agent that reduces the sensitivity of nerves. Valerian root acts as a natural tranquilizer. Turmeric relieves pain since it possesses anti-inflammatory properties. It also prevents blood clots and improves blood circulation. Its active ingredient is curcumin. Curcumin is the main ingredient against inflammation. Turmeric has been used to relieve arthritis pain. Turmeric is also effective against heartburn.

Cloves are effective natural remedies for colds. Cloves also relieve nausea, headaches, arthritic pain and toothaches. Eugenol is the active ingredient in cloves. This active ingredient is found in clove oil. Clove oil is used on an aching tooth until you visit a dentist. Too much of undiluted clove oil may hurt your gums. A dentist's approach is necessary.

Chapter 27
Health Benefits of Aloe

Aloe Vera has a myriad of benefits. It has been used for centuries as a cosmetic means to beauty, but it also heals wounds in the mouth, burns both radiation, (thermal) and skin burns. It gets rid of plaque on teeth.

Aloe has antiseptic properties, anti-tumor effects, a laxative, a moisturizer, treats fungal diseases, hypertension and diabetes mellitus. Clinical trials have been done, and many others are currently underway. The case reports and anecdotal evidence supports all the cosmetic claims and the health benefits. Aloe is a short plant with serrated edges on the leaves. The leaves are triangular, green and succulent. The flowers are tubular and yellow.

Each leaf has three parts: An aloe leaf contains a thick outer layer which serves as the rind and protects the leaf from the environmental factors. It also has a latex layer with a bitter sap that is yellow. This layer acts as the laxative. According to researchers, it has glycosides and anthraquinones. The third part is a clear gel-like liquid with 99% water and vitamins, amino acids, sterols, lipids and glucomannans (sugars).

Aloe Vera contains sugars such as fructose and glucomannans and a glycoprotein, aprogen, with anti-allergenic properties and C-glucosyl Chromone which is an anti-inflammatory compound. Aloe Vera is an antioxidant because it contains minerals that enable the proper functioning of various enzymes in metabolic pathways. Some minerals are antioxidants such as copper, selenium, and zinc which are all found in Aloe Vera.

Aloe also contains vitamin A, C, and E, which are antioxidants and help to keep the skin looking young by neutralizing free radicals. Anthraquinones act as laxatives. Aloe also has analgesic properties. Aloe is rich in bradykinase enzyme, which reduces inflammation. The presence of gibberellins and auxins hormones in Aloe Vera promote anti-inflammation and enhance wound healing processes. Aloe contains a chemical called saponin that has antimicrobial properties.

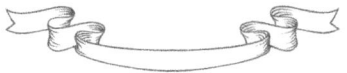

ALOE VERA HAS BEEN proven to possess the following qualities. Aloe Vera promotes collagen synthesis which covers up wounds when the glucomannans and the gibberellin hormone interact with the body's growth hormone. Aloe contains salicylic acid, sulfur, Lupeol and other chemicals that have inhibitory properties on microbes. It stimulates the immune system, and the anthraquinones present inactivates some enveloped viruses.

Aloe enhances the production of fibroblasts which in turn produce elastin and collagen fibers which reduce wrinkling and keeps the skin firm and elastic creating the desired youthful look. Aloe has Anthraquinones that increase intestinal peristalsis, enables mucous secretions and increases the water content in the intestines. The isolation of the anti-inflammatory compound, C- glucosyl Chromone is evidence to the anti-inflammatory properties of Aloe. Aloe Vera also inhibits the production of Arachidonic acid which is responsible for inflammation.

Aloe Vera gel is reported to protect the skin against radiation damage caused by UV rays and Gamma rays to the skin. Aloe Vera stimulates a chemical process that initiates an immune system attack on tumor cells.

Aloe Vera is hailed as a chief herb due to the evidence as mentioned earlier- based health benefits. It is a trusted herbal medication since it produces results over a broad scope of health niches.

Chapter 28

Home Remedies: Science-Backed

Herbs have been in use for centuries. Since now there is herbal medicine, a type of alternative medicine, research is being done to establish the efficacy of these herbs. Some of the herbs under scientific research include the following.

Ginseng is useful for controlling bowel movement, aiding proper digestion and soothing stomach upsets. When used as a tea, it is valuable in controlling coughs, colds and chest infections. It is also an aphrodisiac. Cinnamon is good for soothing stomach upsets, the gas that causes bloating and diarrhea. It promotes healthy blood circulation. Alfalfa is also called Lucerne. It is planted by westerners as cattle fodder, but it is known as a healing herb by Arabs. It is effective against cancer and heart diseases. It is rich in nutrients. It is also rich in minerals. It also relieves constipation, reduces bladder inflammation, reduces bloating and relieves rheumatic pain and cystitis.

The aloe plant has a bitter tasting clear gel. The gel is good for soothing burns. It helps in treating sunburns and thermal burns. When ingested, the extract aims to manage ulcers and any other intestinal anomaly. Too much aloe will act as a laxative when ingested. Angelica root is also known as wild celery, and it's good for treating fevers and colds. Young succulent stems and leaves can be put in a salad. Oregano has been used as an antimicrobial agent. It is applied topically on wounds to prevent infection and promote faster healing processes. It is also a disinfectant and has been used to manage flu and colds. Oregano oil is used to disinfect the room of a sick person.

Garlic possesses anti-inflammatory properties. It is effective in managing inflammation related ailments such as Asthma and cardiovascular illnesses. It is also an antimicrobial agent effective against bacterial and viral infections, as well as boosts immunity. Chamomile is a calming tea. It is good for digestion. It relieves back and treats sunburns and other skin anomalies.

Eucalyptus is used for aroma therapeutic purposes. It is used to remove phlegm in the airways. It also soothes rheumatic pain and stiffness due to arthritis. Peppermint/Mint is used for handling indigestion, eliminating heart burns and nausea. Tea tree oil is used to manage fungal infections topically and other skin diseases. Chlorella is a type of algae that provides protein for vegetarians. Spirulina is also similar to this alga. Caraway seeds aid in increasing breast milk supply. It also used in bringing up phlegm in colds. It helps in digestion as well.

Fennel seeds are used to flavor medicine and food. It also increases menstrual flow and urine volume. It is effective against colic, gout and stomach acidity. It is also an excellent eye wash. It is effective on insect bites, snake bites. It removes an obstruction in the gallbladder, liver, and the spleen. Cloves control nausea and vomiting. It is also used to manage toothaches. Dong Quai is an herb that is available as a supplement. It is suitable for reducing cramps associated with menses. It also controls blood pressure. The elderberry herb has been used to manage neuralgia, colds, and influenza. It is also an excellent blood cleanser. It is used to manage all types of skin infections. It reduces inflammation and controls twitching eyelids.

Echinacea is used to monitor colds and flu. It eliminates Candida infections. It boosts the immune system. It is applied on aching teeth and soothes sore throats. Also used on skin wounds and snake bites. Ginkgo Biloba is also known as maidenhair tree. It possesses anti-inflammatory properties. It is also an antihistamine. It is effective in managing asthma and hemorrhoids. It also boosts circulation, and it improves mental function. It is used to control Alzheimer's disease.

Lemongrass is used as a detoxifier. Lemon balm is effective in treating colic and gas. It is also effective in treating sores around the mouth.

Lemon is an excellent detoxifier. It also prevents scurvy. Thyme possesses antifungal properties. It is used as a cough syrup. Thyme also possesses disinfecting properties. It treats headaches and manages stomach cramps and bowel gas. Vervain is excellent in expelling phlegm build up. It handles common cold infections. It is also used to treat pneumonia and Asthma. Ginger is used to restore appetite. It is also effective in managing nausea. Many more herbs are being studied because they have consistently proven to be effective.

If there is any doubt about the efficacy of these herbs, the scientific studies and related articles in databases such as www.ncbi.nlm.nih.gov can be used to provide adequate scientific information regarding these herbs.

Chapter 29

Headache Relief

Herbs have medicinal value. They relieve pain, clear clogged ENT system and therefore calm any associated symptoms such as headaches. Headaches may be one way that the body tries to communicate to you that something is not right.

You may have a deficiency in a particular vitamin or mineral thus you experience a headache. Allergies also initiate headaches. If you become ill, the body may respond by allowing a headache to ruin your day. Colds, flu and respiratory infections exhibit headaches as a symptom.

Headache Triggers

The following situations may trigger headaches.

1. Allergies

2. Stress

3. Illnesses, e.g., colds and flu

4. Deficiencies in the body

5. Imbalances (Hormonal, Vitamin, and Mineral)

6. Dehydration

7. Hereditary Factors (Certain genes that run in the family)

Essential oils and herbs relieve headaches. Not all herbs relieve pain, but the ones that do, have a high success rate. There are no side effects when using herbs. This is an advantage in today's world where many people are trying to stay healthy. Medication and pills for headache relief usually cause a deficiency elsewhere in the body leading to a cycle of painkiller dependence.

For instance, Magnesium in low levels will result in a headache and painkillers that deplete magnesium in the body may relieve a particular headache at the expense of your future health. Sooner or later, you will end up having a more severe headache because the body is trying to signal you of a shortage in magnesium. This cycle creates a health crisis that herbs do not create. The following herbs will not cause repeat headaches. They have been reputed as effective headache remedies.

Lavender has sedative properties. It also enhances good moods. It relieves headaches especially the ones associated with Migraines. Migraine headaches are usually hereditary. They have no underlying cause just faulty genes. Peppermint essential oil is good for relieving tension associated headaches. It is also effective on headaches caused by stress or a heavy workout at the gym. Peppermint produces a cooling effect on the skin causing tension in muscles to dissipate. It is the source for menthol. Menthol unblocks clogged respiratory systems and blocked noses due to colds and flu. Therefore, it is effective against illness caused headaches.

Feverfew herb is also effective against migraines. It relieves the symptoms that are associated with this type of headache such as light sensitivity. It also reduces sensitivity to sounds. Noise increases migraine longevity. Feverfew reduces the sensitivity to noise and loud sounds. Feverfew herb also curbs nausea and vomiting bouts. Butterbur herb is a natural beta blocker. It inhibits any chemicals causing inflammation from being released. It is effective on migraines.

Ginger is a naturally occurring anti-inflammatory agent. It helps to reduce tension in muscles and blood vessels. This allows for proper blood circulation. It can be added to water when trying to beat dehydration. It works on any headaches triggered by dehydration when ingested with water. Also useful for allergy related headache since it acts against inflammation. Allergens cause inflammation which is known as an allergy. Since lemon is known for its excellent cleansing properties, it relieves headaches when the body metabolism works fine as a result of toxin removal through cleansing. It is useful against any headaches associated with hormonal imbalances and Vitamin C deficiencies.

Mint Juice is extracted from the leaves of the herb and applied on the temples and the forehead. The soothing effect of the menthol in the juice relieves headaches. Basil is a natural analgesic. It is also calming and relaxes tense muscles. The leaves can be chewed or made into an herbal tea. Basil oil can also be massaged on the temples. Cayenne Pepper is a medicinal herb. It is used as a spice for that chili effect on meals. Apart from being a spice, one health benefit is its ability to cure headaches. It improves blood flow by acting on the vein structure. It treats intestinal ulcers, rectifies stomach muscles and reduces high blood pressure. Since it corrects symptoms of illnesses, it relieves any associated headaches. Inhaling the smell of crushed cloves relieves headaches associated with allergies since cloves have anti-inflammatory properties. It gives immediate pain relief and produces a cooling effect when inhaled. Going herbal instead of popping pills will keep you out of the hospital in the long run. The probability of getting a drug induced mineral deficiency is little to none.

Chapter 30
Herbal Teas

Herbal tea is not tea. It is a combination of leaves, bark, fruit, and other extracts of a particular herb. The herb is known for its medicinal and healing properties. Herbs are known to soothe insomnia, calm nerves in the case of anxiety disorders, relieve a bloated stomach, and help ease sleep abnormalities.

Herbal tea can be ingested with the aim of getting the full medicinal value or as a stimulant. Herbal tea is a healthy tonic to get enough sleep, which comes quickly, they also aid in aromatherapy while being ingested, and bowel movement to soothe an aching stomach. Medicinal values include relief from a sore throat, bronchitis, and fever. Some herbal teas act against cancers and diseases of the heart. Other herbal teas are detoxifiers in nature and help in body cleansing purposes.

Lemon extracts are usually best served at room temperature. Serving lemon tea at room temperature allows the body to get all the benefits of vitamin C that are found in lemons. It is also claimed that frozen lemons, when grated over water with the rind intact, is helpful in relieving cancer symptoms, an excellent detoxifier and a great cleanser.

Chickweed Tea grows as a weed in many gardens. It can be made into a soothing hot drink when ground into powder, fresh from the garden or dried. Its health benefits are not affected as much as lemon tea. This herb has medicinal properties of soothing colic, coughs, bronchitis and many issues arising from the respiratory system.

Ginger herbal tea is known to soothe the digestive system. It is used to relieve an upset stomach and curb nausea. It is also used to stop headaches arising from common colds. Used as an aromatherapy asset to unblock stuffy noses as a result of flu. Ginger tea is also good for relieving morning sickness.

Green tea used for detoxification purposes, and since it keeps free radicals from affecting aging, you are guaranteed to have that youthful look on your skin. It also reduces the risk of cancer. Rosehip tea herbal tea is made from the fruits of the rose plant. The fruits are rich in vitamin C. The advantage of this tea over lemon tea is that while heat will make it lose some nutrients, higher amounts for the body are retained in hot water.

Eucalyptus tea is probably the best aroma therapeutic agent in this chapter. It is an herbal tea, but with additional therapy for the nose. It is useful in unblocking stuffy noses, and clearing phlegm that is blocking the respiratory tract. It is also an anti-inflammatory agent in relieving rheumatic, and arthritis that induces swelling. The aroma therapeutic benefits induce calmness and a good night's sleep, especially during common cold infections and flu.

Chapter 31
Olive Leaf for Better Health

Olive leaf has seen a great action in the human diet, where it has been used as an extract, powder as well as herbal tea for years. The leaf is preferred for its bioactive compounds as rich in antioxidants, anti-atherogenic, antihypertensive, and anti-inflammatory. It is also known for its hypoglycemic and hypocholesterolemic qualities. Well, here are top nine benefits you can get from olive leaf.

According to study, olive leaf is effective in reducing both systolic and diastolic blood pressure. Besides, this leaf is effective in reducing bad cholesterol (triglycerides) in the body and does not come with most side effects like a dry cough, dizziness or loss of taste that could result from the use of other treatments like captopril.

Olive leaf is one of the cardiovascular function boosters used for centuries as an herbal tonic. Its extract has proved efficient in lowering excessive levels of LDL cholesterol as well as maintaining the blood pressure. Thanks to glycosides Oleuropein and its product hydroxytyrosol, is crucial for reducing coronary heart disease and treating some cancers. The olive leaf extract has also proved to reverse cardiovascular stress as well as chronic inflammation, which is responsible for causing several diseases.

What's more, the hyperglycemic effects of this extract help reduce the body's blood sugar levels besides controlling blood glucose levels. Then it plays yet another important role, as its polyphenols assist in preventing the production of sugar from consuming starch, which could otherwise lead to diabetes and other diseases caused by inflammatory. Another vital importance of olive leaves is that these are a natural treatment for several cancer types. Since it is capable of stopping the angiogenic process that stimulates tumor growth, the leaves are essential for keeping cancer at bay. Besides, it also features the compound oleuropein, which has the necessary antioxidant and anti-angiogenic capabilities for suppressing the development and spread of advanced tumors. According to one study, olive leaves can help prevent breast cancer, urinary bladder cancer as well as cancer of the brain. Olive leaf also packs a great deal for the function of our brain. According to another study, the oleuropein in these leaves helps reduce age-related disorders like Alzheimer's disease and dementia. This is thanks to the leaves' antioxidants, which help fight effects caused by free radicals that interfere with memory loss. The use of olive leaf as an extract or infusion offers a natural treatment for Alzheimer's diseases among other brain problems.

Arthritis causes pain and swelling in the joints, which can be attributed to inflammation. But olive leaf anti-inflammatory properties make it ideal for treating this problem as a natural remedy. A study conducted in 2012 indicated that these leaves could treat paw swelling due to arthritis. Research has also shown that the leaves help reduce pain related to osteoarthritis as well as reducing cytokines production and the inflammation-causing enzymes.

Another great thing about olive leaf is the ability to treat infections like candida, pneumonia, chronic fatigue, meningitis, pneumonia, malaria, hepatitis B, gonorrhea, and tuberculosis, as well as shingles. Moreover, this is an ideal natural treatment for dental problems, ear infection, and infections in the urinary tract. The leaves also help kill bacteria like dermatophytes, responsible for causing skin, nails and hair disease. They are also ideal for fighting candida albicans that cause oral and genital infection, as well as fighting Escherichia coli cells, the bacteria that reside in the lower intestine.

Olive leaves are high in antiviral properties, which make it ideal for preventing serious threats like viruses to the mild ones like a common cold. From influenza-causing viruses to other infections in the respiratory system, these leaves are efficient for the body's defense. Thanks to potent compounds capable of destroying invading organisms, and preventing viruses from multiplying and treating infections, olive leaves are ideal when it comes to keeping your body safe.

If your skin is damaged, olive leaf can still reverse the effect and wear out any signs of aging, thanks to its antioxidant properties that help inhibit cell damage from oxidation. According to study, skin damage from UV radiation leads to low skin elasticity and thickness, telltale signs of skin damage. Olive leaf comes in handy in the treatment of the problem, and further inhibits carcinogenesis and tumor growth in the skin. You can always get a broad range of advantages with olive leaf extracts.

Chapter 32
Papaya Leaf Extract

In the quest for health supplements and herbal remedies, the conventional options are becoming sidelined day after day. Apparently, as much as organic foods are taking the cake, the food type is also devoid of nutrients. When it comes to the nutrient content, food used decades ago had much to offer than most current types, which means the need for even more options to get the best possible nutrient from the food available.

As soils are depleted and most of the available vitamins offering little benefits to go by, additional supplements are becoming popular by the day. Some of the leading ones include turmeric, cacao, vitamin D and some other essential supplements that have proved crucial for better health. Well, papaya leaf extract is one of the most sought-after supplements, and for good reasons.

ONE THING REMAINS CLEAR; supplements are taking center stage in offering incredible health. But why is papaya gaining popularity as an ideal solution to boost your health? Well, this plant is high in essential elements for a healthy body, like Vitamin A, Vitamin E, Vitamin C, dietary fiber and foliates among others. Besides, papaya is also rich in antioxidants, carotenoids, and flavonoids, which add to the plant's incredible benefits when it comes to attaining unprecedented health.

And there is more; this plant further packs a good level of an enzyme papain, as well as chymopapain. These enzymes are necessary for the health of your body, as enzymes go a long way in helping the control of both physical and mental functions, which are essential for life and health.

Most important of all, you need to understand the actual uses of papaya and the benefits of this plant. Papaya has been used for centuries, thanks to its advantages, and now its leaf extract is bringing back the glory with some outstanding healing properties. These uses and benefits include the following:

• Support for the cardiovascular as well as gastrointestinal systems.

• Boost to immunity system.

• It also helps break down proteins and production of digestive enzymes, which is crucial for the digestive system.

• The extract also helps with the renewal of muscle tissue and increasing the quality of proteins in organisms.

• Besides, papaya leaf also helps with revitalizing and maintenance of energy and vitality in the human body.

• What's more, this is also an effective treatment for skin wounds and prevention of cataract, not to mention eliminating constipation and nausea.

• Above all, the extract is also essential for the treatment of cancers of different types, and you can count on its high vitamin D level for lowering emphysema in smokers.

Perhaps the best part about this extract is that it offers not only ideal treatment for gastrointestinal tract and help with digestive problems, but also provides many more health benefits. From the benefits discussed above to others like the use of papaya enzyme in eliminating parasites in the body, you can always get more with this extract.

Chapter 33
Soursop Leaf Benefits for Your Health

Soursop is a native fruit of South America, Southeast Asia, and Africa, which is also known as graviola. The evergreen plant has broad leaves useful for medicine, and its fruit has a sweet-sour taste with a sweet aroma. But what has seen this plant become popular is its ability to fight cancer as well as some other medicinal properties as well.

Forget chemotherapy and other contemporary cancer treatment options that could end in disastrous side effects. This plant packs qualities for killing cancer cells, and it has proved to be more than ten thousand times more potent than chemotherapy according to research. In fact, the plant is robust for treating different notorious cancers like lung cancer, breast cancer, and prostate cancer.

Soursop leaves are also popular for treating gout, which has seen it become used as the most reliable alternative medicine for this condition. All you need to do is intake around six to ten leaves, wash them and boil in two cups of water, then let simmer to retain one cup. Take the concoction two times daily until you see results.

Back pain is becoming endemic these days, especially during exercise. But the use of chemicals to deal with back pain could lead to unwanted side effects, and a natural remedy comes in handy here. Soursop leaves never disappoint, and all you need is about twenty leaves of the plant boiled in five cups of water and simmered to retain only three cups. Take ¾ cup once every day.

Rheumatic disease is common in seniors, and responsible for causing extreme pain. If arthritis is becoming a serious problem, then soursop leaves offer an ideal natural remedy. Smash them until smooth and apply on the affected area, preferably twice daily. For the average blood sugar, the range should be anywhere between 70 and 120 milligrams, but in case of any changes, soursop leaves can come to your rescue. These leaves can stabilize the level of sugar in this range, and thus help as a natural treatment for diabetes.

The other benefit you will come to love about these leaves is the ability to enhance your immune system to keep infections at bay. To achieve this, you only need to boil about 4/5 leaves in four cups of water and simmer to have one cup remain, than drink the concoction once daily to get the preferred results.

From bacteria to viruses, parasites, and development of tumors, these leaves have numerous benefits. Besides, these leaves are used for anti-seizure medication, lowering high blood pressure, boils and treating fever as well. You can also count on these leaves for treatment of swollen feet or inflammation, aiding in digestion problems as well as improving appetite. Above all, if you take these leaves on a daily basis, you can enhance your stamina and facilitate quick recovery in case of diseases.

Chapter 34
Dietary Treatments for Anemia

A nemia may not be a cause to freak you out, but this could be bad news for a serious illness in your body. It is, therefore, necessary to consult your doctor to be sure the type of anemia, whether it is sickle cell, hemolytic, or sideroblastic anemia. Such anemia types result from a malfunction in the body, a situation that can be contained by medical means. However, in normal health conditions, anemia could be a sign of deficiency in nutrition, like lack of iron, folic acid or Vitamin B12. If you have anemia from nutritional deficiency, there are several remedies to use at home.

Apples are high in iron and come with several other healthy components too. On its side, beet is rich in folic acid, potassium, and fiber. The most nutritious part is right on the peel, so cooking while still unpeeled and removing the skin later could help. You may have more than one apple in a day, but the combination of beet and apples give you a better edge.

Blackstrap molasses not only pack a high amount of iron but also are also rich in folate that offers an ideal source of folic acid. Besides, they come with sufficient amounts of Vitamin B. the combination of these elements make molasses a great deal for fighting anemia, and anyone who has diabetes can take advantage of the low glycemic index in molasses.

You can treat anemia with a half a cup of spinach per day, thanks to the green's high levels of Vitamin A, C, B9, and E, as well as calcium, fiber, beta-carotene, and iron. Hence, including this vegetable in your daily diet could go the distance in keeping anemia at bay. But spinach contains oxalic acid, which inhibits uptake of iron, but boiling the leaves can reduce the acid level.

Pomegranate fruit has many benefits, from proteins, fat, fiber, carbohydrates, and sugar. It is also high in essential minerals like copper, potassium and a good number of vitamins as well. This fruit increases blood hemoglobin levels and helps attain the right flow of blood, leading to reduced exhaustion, weakness, dizziness, and other symptoms of anemia.

If you do not have these remedies handy in your home, you can also try other viable options. From parsley, raisins, and whole grains, there is much to go around when it comes to anemia fighting remedies. Besides, legumes, nuts, ash gourd and bottle gourd are as helpful too. Not forgetting, yellow dock herbal decoction and wheat germ iron tonic, as well as the ideal diet planning, goes a long way. It is also worth considering which option offers a high amount of iron, especially if your levels are dropping fast.

Chapter 35
Herbs to Control Cystitis

Infection of the urinary tract can prove fatal even on a one time deal, but the sad part is, this condition will most likely hit again. And whenever it comes back, the situation worsens. In essence, this problem leads to distressing symptoms like lower abdomen pain, urgent or frequent need to pass urine as well as a feeling of burning sensation when someone disposes of urine. It is also possible to see blood in the urine.

Bacteria cause cystitis, so the use of antibiotics usually treats it. However, some of the bacteria might survive in this kind of treatment, resulting in a repeat of the infection. Besides, the antibiotic treatment could pose the threat of unwanted side effects like allergy reactions on skin, thrush, diarrhea, and vomiting among others.

The bacteria can remain dormant for some time, but it could become active under several factors. These could include causes like diabetes, menopause, using spermicides, sexual intercourse or changes in the acid-forming bacteria in the vagina. If this happens, someone could suffer from infections that are recurrent, but using the right herbs could become a preventive treatment.

Cranberry herb is one of the most useful measures in fighting cystitis. Some of the bacteria that cause this condition like E. coli use tiny projections to hang on to the bladder. So this herb is essential in preventing the bacteria from clinging to the walls. Thus, it is reliable in eliminating the bacteria present and any chances of recurrent infections.

Bearberry contains arbutin, a phytochemical that can help in fighting bacteria. Bacteria in the urine can convert this chemical into hydroquinone, which has high potency for killing the harmful bacteria. This means the herb helps the bacteria produce their own toxin. You should take 3 grams a day in case of acute cystitis and half the dose in case of recurrent one.

Besides these herbs, others also go a long way in preventing the effects of these bacteria from taking hold. These include buchu and juniper, which also act as antibacterial agents in the urine. The other options you can turn to include Echinacea, which is potent for prevention of this disease, and Andrographis, which helps treat acute cystitis. For instance, Echinacea root or the use of Ayurvedic herb can be far-reaching in supporting your immune system to keep infection at bay.

Remember, you need to keep on taking these herbs even if the symptoms decline. You can continue with the dose for about three to four months, just to be sure there are no chances of any remaining bacteria in your urinary bladder. Besides, you should watch on your diet, primarily by consuming cranberry and drinking up to eight glasses of water daily to flush out the bugs. It is also essential to reduce your intake of sugary foods or refined carbs like pasta and white bread to prevent accumulation of sugar in your urine. Eating more green veggies and high protein foods to enhance your immune system could also become beneficial. Above all, consider wearing loose underwear and go for the cotton material to lower the risk of irritation. And while bathing may increase the chances of bacteria reaching your urethra from the phallus, a shower could be the best option.

Chapter 36
Herbs for Fighting Plaque

In essence, plaque forms and develops inside the arteries, cause clogging, and hardening of blood vessels. The development of this problem could lead to strokes or heart attacks due to lack of blood supply to vital organs. These clots result from sticky platelets and plaque from the walls of artery could block blood flow with serious effects, even death. But this problem does not have to take a toll on your health; you can count on these seven herbs.

Hawthorn has been essential in the treatment of cardiovascular diseases. This herb is used in doses of between 160 and 1,800 mg daily. It is also potent in preventing the formation of plaque in the arteries as well as reducing blood pressure and lowering cholesterol levels as well. Hawthorn has polyphenols known as quercetin and rutin. Besides, it comes with antioxidant properties that help in preventing plaque buildup and improving cardiovascular health.

Turmeric contains compounds like curcumin, which can help prevent blood platelets from coagulating. The compound further helps in getting rid of formation of plaque in the arteries. This herb was used in Traditional Chinese Medicine to invigorate the blood. The herbs potent antioxidant action prevents oxidation of LDL cholesterol, which helps lower blood cholesterol levels.

Psyllium comprises of some soluble fiber and can help reduce cholesterol, which is a principal causative agent of plaque. Psyllium has also proved to reduce cholesterol as well as blood triglyceride levels. Apart from lowering cholesterol levels, the herb also comes in handy in lowering blood sugar.

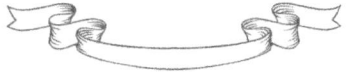

HORNY GOAT WEED WAS used formerly in treating hardening arteries as well as other symptoms associated with the disease. According to a study by University of Michigan Health System, it improves symptoms as well as helping people with hardening of arteries through an electrocardiogram.

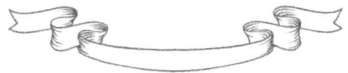

GINGER IS YET ANOTHER viable option when it comes to fighting this problem. Taking a given amount of the herb per day helps prevent stickiness in platelets as well as clearing arteries with any traces of plaque. The best part is that whether dry or fresh, the herb helps manipulate platelets. It comes with more than twelve antioxidants that help reduce the levels of cholesterol in the serum while still improving circulation and preventing the risk of blood clotting in the arteries.

Garlic is among the best herbs you can count on in preventing blood clot build up inside arteries. You can take this herb as a capsule, although the fresh garlic can also be useful. Garlic helps lower cholesterol levels to prevent such clots and keep plaque at bay. Besides, this herb can help women seeking to prevent or treat atherosclerosis. This is thanks to components in the herb like allicin and constituent ajoene, which prevent blood clots forming or blood platelets sticking. The other benefit is this herb can aid in preventing oxidation of LDL cholesterol, also known as bad cholesterol, especially when consumed as the old extract. If you want to prevent aggregation of the blood platelets, Bilberry is hands down the go-to option. This herb thus comes in handy in preventing clots and plaque formation, according to the University of Michigan Health System. The herb has also shown positive effects on the contraction of the heart as well as blood vessels.

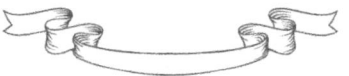

ALTHOUGH GUGGUL HAS shown mixed results in its effects depending on the time of consumption, this herb is effective in lowering cholesterol levels. The herb is also useful in preventing plaque from building up in arteries. Guggul has also proved to be potent in avoiding cholesterol in people who usually eat traditionally low-fat foods.

Chapter 37
Stress Reducing Herbs

S tress can take a toll on your peace of mind, and sometimes even your health too. It is thus essential to ensure you keep the dangerous predicament at bay for as long as you can, and herbs could be one of the best ways to do so. Perhaps the best part is that you can make the most of the numerous natural herbs as well as supplements available to reduce stress without risking side effects.

Passionflower herb is hands down one of the best options for people with increased levels of anxiety. It is known to help them attain good sleep, and it is famous as an aphrodisiac in the old Polynesian cultures. It has mild sedative effects, but not as soft as the Valerian though.

Ashwagandha, also known as the winter cherry has been used for years, helping in soothing the mind in case of agitation. The herb's roots are high in flavonoids as well as high levels of withanolide class. Since it is an adaptogen, it helps the user adapt to different environments, which can work pretty well for the stressful situations too. If you have problems sleeping, the soothing scent of Lavender will aid in this case. And if you can laugh enough and have a good time to unwind from a long, terrible day, you should consider smelling this flower. You can as well drink tea infused with the herb for an instant calm feeling if you have frazzled nerves.

Magnesium supplements or taking food rich in this mineral could help soothe tight and sore muscles. But it does not end there; Magnesium is also renowned for its ability to reduce blood pressure and lower stress levels. Besides, the mineral is useful for lowering anomalies in the heartbeat as well as keeping the cardiovascular system working correctly. And if you have type 2 diabetes; insomnia, or depression, this mineral will work well for you.

Chamomile herb can be taken as a supplement or merely brew it in a tea. Aiding in calming nerves and easing the mind, it's mildly sedating properties come in handy for people who can't sleep so quickly due to stress. According to research on its performance, especially for people with anxiety disorders, the herb proven to work pretty well than placebos if taken daily. With Kava you can brew the roots of this herb to create a drink ideal for calming down anxiety. Besides, it comes with sedative properties, which help in feeling better without necessarily interrupting your cognition. Its uses include treating social anxiety over the perilous alcoholic drinks choice.

Green and black teas have L-theanine, which increases the alpha waves in the brain as well as helping attain a feeling of calmness. According to studies, L-theanine lowers the level of harmful approach to stress, and it has proved to increase relaxation in people who have critical behavioral disorders.

Chapter 38
Uses of Hemp

Hemp is naturally a fiber, which also happens to be a cousin of the cannabis sativa. The plant has been used for industrial purposes over the years, and it not only offers environment-friendly products. Besides, it can as well be used in jewelry, food, fuels, clothing, and many more uses as well. Hemp has a long history, and humankind has been using it for all types of functions. The use of hemp in textile includes the making of clothes, shoes, hats, as well as accessories. The plant has proved useful in this way for decades, and this is all thanks to its absorbent, warm and durable natural fibers. Besides, the plant can be grown in areas where cotton cannot thrive, since it is resistant to weather and moisture, and it is cost-effective in production. The versatility of the plant means it can be blended with other types of fibers like cotton and silk, which adds to its extensive use for this purpose.

Another impressive aspect of this plant is that it can help as an environment-friendly replacement for gasoline. The plant burns clean, producing methanol. These hydrocarbons are renewable and can assist in attaining fuel without polluting the atmosphere. Moreover, the fiber, as well as seeds, is used as biomass fuel, not to mention that it offers a great deal of ethanol and biodiesel as well.

The other interesting use of this plant is in the manufacture of body products like shampoo, massage oils, conditioners, skin crèmes, sunscreens, soaps, and lotions, to mention but a few. First, the plant is a safe alternative when it comes to looking for the ideal ingredient with the least chance of causing an allergic reaction. Moreover, it is renowned for its abilities to treat dermatitis and several other conditions of the skin, not forgetting that hemp is a green ingredient without harsh chemicals or toxins that could damage the skin. Besides the industrial use, hemp is an ideal ingredient when it comes to getting the best value for our health. The plant's seeds are high in vegetable protein, which ranks them as second to soybeans. But the best part is that these are easily digestible. Besides, you don't need to cook and ferment it to be able to eat it, and it tastes good nevertheless. The plant is incorporated in such foods as cheese, cake mixes, peanut butter, crackers and much more.

Besides, hemp offers numerous proteins useful in pet food as well. For your small household animals like cats, dogs, to the bigger ones like horses and cows, chicken, and several other bird species, hemp offers something for everyone. Rich in Vitamin A among other benefits, the plant provides the best for your pets as it does for all of your family.

Hemp has been used extensively for commercial purposes, offering a broad range of products for customer use. From fabrics to biomass fuel, biodegradable products, and body care products as well as detergents, wood, paper and food products to mention but a few.

Chapter 39
Herbal Remedies for Varicose Veins

People suffer from multiple blood circulation problems, and varicose veins are one of the most frustrating conditions you may have to treat. Cayenne pepper is high in flavonoids and Vitamin C. These help prevent free radical damage to blood vessel walls as well as enhancing formation of collagen to keep these walls elastic and healthy. What's more, cayenne comes with capsaicin, which is potent with an anti-inflammatory, blood thinning properties, as well as analgesic. Powder from this herb can help prevent blood clotting and ulcers as well.

Grape Seed extract is derived from tiny seeds in grapes, which have antioxidant substances like flavonoids, Vitamin E, and linoleic acid among others. The extract also packs potent vasoprotective qualities. It is responsible for preventing damage to blood vessel walls from free radicals and promotes the formation of collagen. This is a protein useful for maintaining elastic properties of connective tissues as well as improving the strength of walls in blood vessels. Above all, it guards against leakage of fluid from veins and subsequent swelling in legs.

Pine bark extract contains flavonoids, phenolic acids, and proanthocyanidins, all which help reduce varicose veins and the inflammation caused by this problem. When taken orally, the extract helps strengthen walls of blood vessels and binds the protein collagen to redeem elasticity. It also improves circulation and reduces pressure to ease leg cramps and pain resulting from standing for long. Horse chestnut can be extracted from the leaves, bark, seeds, or flowers of Aesculus hippocastanum, a plant that is renowned for treating this problem and other circulatory diseases as well. It has Aescin, a vasoprotective agent responsible for suppressing the enzymes that damage blood vessel walls. Aescin offers an astringent quality, which causes constriction or shrinking of body tissues like blood vessels and others.

Besides, the extract helps with blood thinning, which enhances circulation while eliminating the chances of blood clotting that could lead to varicose veins. Not forgetting, it has an anti-inflammatory effect as well as a diuretic action for reducing pain or swelling in the affected area. You can apply it on any ulcers on your leg, but do not ingest it or use it to brew tea, as it is toxic. Keep in mind that this remedy is not ideal for people with bleeding problems and pregnant women.

Pot marigold works with virtually any type of skin problem, although this may not treat varicose veins directly. But in case of eczema, dryness, ulcers, itching or such skin conditions, preparing an infusion of this herb's petals in boiling water and pressing it on the area could help. Besides, you can soak it in a warm bath, and add flowers for effect. Its anti-inflammatory properties help reduce pain and inflammation, not to mention that it restores the natural skin texture through promoting collagens. Other types of herbs to turn to if you have this kind of problem include Gotu Kola, Apple cider vinegar, and chamomile oil. All these can be very helpful in fighting the effects of varicose veins on your legs.

Chapter 40
Herbs for Cleansing your Lungs and Respiratory System

Did you know that your respiratory is not only one of the most critical systems that keep you alive? But while this is your lifeline, it can be one of the areas prone to the entrance of irritants, mold, dust, fungus, and other pollutants and toxins. So, how do you keep your lungs and the entire respiratory system safe from this menace? There is good news; nature offers some of the essential herbs as well as botanicals that you can take advantage of for the nutrition of your respiratory system. Oregano has many benefits for the body, with nutrients and vitamins. But it is renowned for its rosmarinic and carvacrol acid, which help as natural decongestants and reducing histamine. These are beneficial to the respiratory tract as well as the nasal cavity air passage. Besides, carvacrol helps boost the body's immune system as well.

Lungwort herb aids in promoting healthy lungs as well as respiratory system health. It also helps clear congestion. Its effectiveness comes from potent compounds, which fight harmful organisms that can be a threat to the respiratory system. Chaparral is a native of the southwest and is famous for its detoxification effect on the lungs as well as respiratory support. It is rich in potent antioxidants that prevent irritation as well as possessing NDGA, which is helpful in fighting histamine response. Moreover, the herb helps counter harmful organisms. It can be used as chaparral tea or tincture extraction.

Eucalyptus offers a refreshing aroma and promotes respiratory system health as well as soothing irritation in the throat. The plant is also widely used as an ingredient in syrups and cough lozenges. It offers an adequate remedy to several problems thanks to a compound cineole, which helps in easing coughing, fighting congestion, as well as soothing irritation in the sinus passage, not to mention that it is also an expectorant. Besides, the herb's antioxidant properties boost the immune system when you have a cold.

PEPPERMINT, AS WELL as its oil, has menthol that helps as a soothing ingredient for relaxing smooth muscles in the respiratory tract to promote natural breathing. Along with the antihistamine effect that peppermint offers, the menthol also comes in handy as a decongestant. Not forgetting, the herb is also useful in fighting harmful organisms and its antioxidant effects are far reaching as well. Since back in the 1800's, Elecampane herb roots have been the ingredients in cough medicine and lozenges. This helps to aid relaxing effects on the smooth muscle in the trachea. Elecampane has two active compounds, alantolactone, which is an expectorant with anti-tissue action and inulin, which helps soothe bronchial passage.Lobelia herb contains lobeline, an alkaloid that is effective in thinning mucus and breaking up congestion. Besides, Lobelia aids in stimulating adrenal glands to help produce epinephrine, which allows the air passages to relax for more natural breathing.

ACCORDING TO CLINICAL trials, Plantain Leaf has proved to be effective against cold, cough and lung irritation among other respiratory problems. Besides, it can also trigger the production of mucus in the lungs to relieve a dry cough. Osha roots are high in camphor as well as other compounds that have seen this herb become renowned as a crucial lung-support in the medical world. One of the herb's benefits is its effectiveness in boosting circulation in the lungs for more natural breathing.

Chapter 41

Herbs for Hormone Control

Perhaps the best part is that you can take charge of your hormones with natural and potent herbs, which comes without compromising your health. These are known as adaptogens, which help your body adapt to the environment and metabolic changes.

Among the essential things associated with Saw Palmetto is reducing chronic fatigue and improve sperm count. What's more, its berry comes in very handy in the treatment of benign prostatic hyperplasia. This herb also helps in relieving stress as well as improving the immune system. The best part is that this herb can also aid balancing endocrine system effects as well as being active on the reproductive systems of both sexes.

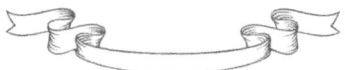

ASHWAGANDHA IS A FAVORITE in Indian medicine Ayurveda, used in manipulating the endocrine system, which makes this herb ideal as an adaptogen by influencing the adrenal glands. It also affects the thyroid, which helps in fighting hyperthyroidism. Ashwagandha can also improve blood circulation, reduce stress, and slow down premature aging among other benefits.

Astragalus usually features in TCM for treatment of various health issues like liver problems, heart and infections in the upper respiratory as well. Currently, Astragalus is also a standard option for stimulating immunity. The most effective part of this herb for hormone control is the fact that it regulates blood pressure as well as sugar levels in the blood. Besides, it is useful for the protection of insulin-secreting beta cells in the pancreas, thus controlling hormone resistance.

American ginseng has a more controlled and milder effect than Chinese ginseng, but it is just as effective. Usually, American ginseng is effective in supporting the axis of hypothalamus-pituitary-adrenal HPA for ideal hormonal balance. The herb strengthens the immune system and helps relieve stress, improving digestion and promoting absorption and assimilation of nutrients among other benefits.

Maca Root is highly nutritious and usually consumed as a vegetable. But its energy boosting properties is what makes it stand out. Besides, its hormone balancing effect offers added advantages like reducing stress among other benefits. Other hormonal control benefits of this root include relief for women with premenstrual syndrome as well as symptoms such as night sweats and hot flashes that are associated with menopause.

Tribulus is primarily considered as an aphrodisiac. Besides, thanks to its ability to stimulate androgen receptors, it helps achieve better utilization of male sex hormones. This, in turn, helps increase sperm count and treat other male reproductive issues as well. Moreover, a component protodioscin in this herb also helps in improving men's DHEA levels, thus boosting erectile function and fertility. These are just some of the exotic herbs that you can use to bring your hormones under control for better health. Other types of herbs include epimedium, chasteberry, Suma root and black cohosh, which are useful in dealing with multiple problems of hormonal balance.

Chapter 42

Acne and Traditional Remedies

In today's world, junk food has become popular, but apparently not ideal for your health. From saturated fat to iodized salt, high-glycemic foods, a contemporary world diet can be your best friend or your worst enemy. Garlic helps relieve pain and improves the healing effect of acne. You can use raw garlic to rub on acne several times per day.

Use basil to make an infusion of the herb's leaves by placing two or four teaspoons in a cup of water heated to a boil for ten to twenty minutes. Let it cool and apply it to acne. If you are looking for an ideal cleanser for your skin, Aloe Vera juice fights infection and helps attain faster healing. Just split the leaf and rub on the surface.

For a potent antimicrobial agent and a disinfectant in one herb, grape seed extract will have you covered. All you need is to prepare a solution of about four to forty drops in water, or equal to four ounces, then apply it on the affected area twice or three times per day.

If you have an acne problem, cleaning your skin and applying lemon juice can help. The acid in this herb flushes the pores for beautiful skin. You can also use steam to wash your face, primarily by putting your face over a pan of boiling lemon water, with a towel over your head to harness the steam. Coriander is used by including it in tea, about 0.5 teaspoons of the herb, fennel, and cumin. Place it in boiling water for ten minutes or so. Drinking after meals would be best. Using chickpea paste to wash your face then drying it with a clean towel offers an excellent remedy for treating acne as well.

Peel cucumber and liquefy it using a blender before applying the juice onto your acne. Besides, you can drink about four or five cups of the herb's juice on a daily basis for one week to purify the lymphatic system and blood for clear skin. Blend beetroot juice and carrot juice, add water. This helps stimulate the liver for cleansing.

Neem is used for Ayurvedic medicine thanks to its healing properties like anti-fungal, anti-bacterial, and antiviral potency. In case of acne, you can take about five fresh leaves in the morning. These herbs are some of the best options when it comes to fighting acne.

Chapter 43
Alkaline Water for Better Health

How often do you drink alkaline water? Probably not every day, but you should from time to time try it. Alkaline water has proved to be useful for people suffering from diabetes, hypertension, high cholesterol, and several other benefits too. The pH level in this water exceeds the level you will find in your regular drinking water, and this is believed to help neutralize body acid. All this comes with a wide range of benefits.

This water not only keeps your skin well hydrated, it further helps fight free radicals that can mean faster aging. This results in better skin health and a younger appearance. If you want a younger looking and glowing complexion, then alkaline water is a great option. Acidity can alter metabolism in the body. This can result in excessive production of acid in the stomach, which can emanate from alcohol, stress, overeating, as well as other factors. These can also cause heartburn due to acid reflux. The addition of alkalizing water in diet and several alkalizing foods helps in neutralizing the effects caused by this acidic nature for better digestion.

Sometimes diets are too acidic that people suffer degradation of the bone density in the aftermath, and probably osteoporosis as well. These results could have lasting consequences in your life. Well, alkaline water can help in neutralizing this acidity in your diet, which can reduce effects such as bone failure from these conditions. Drinking a lot of water can help attain energy, which is the opposite of a weakened, dehydrated body. With alkaline water, you take matters a notch higher as this type of water delivers nutrients essential to the body than ordinary tap water can offer.

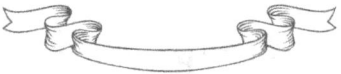

ACCUMULATION OF TOXINS in the body can lead to uncontrolled weight gain and obesity. These toxins are deposited in fat tissues, which can be caused by excessive acidity in the body along with other health problems as well. Using alkaline water helps reduce this acidity to help prevent such storage of excessive fat. Therefore, this water and alkalizing diet can lead to a great deal of weight loss in the long term. With this type of negatively charged water containing antioxidants, you can be sure it will be useful in fighting free radicals. These properties help prevent diseases and slow down your aging process and symptoms like wrinkles and sagging of the skin as well as reducing damage to DNA cells from damage and preventing tissue damage altogether.

Chapter 44

Chinese Herbs in Treating Systemic Lupus Erythematosis SLE

L upus is a disease resulting from antibodies attacking connective tissues. The disease is systematic, although some cases involve discoid lupus and circumscribed forms. This type of condition usually occurs from antinuclear antibodies, which target the nucleic acid guanine, circulation of immune complexes as well as activating complacent systems.

Lupus is mild in most cases, but some severe ones usually occur especially if the condition is not treated in time. This can affect the skin and progress to severe attacks on lungs, kidneys, heart, as well as other organs. The disease manifests in flare-ups that can be triggered by emotional stress, exposure to ultraviolet light, or infections.

The use of immunosuppressive strategies is used in most modern medical treatments, including the use of corticosteroids like prednisone, which is administered if flare-ups manifest. However, despite how effective the procedure may be, the side effects of drugs, along with low-level manifestation of the disease can be drastic.

Some of the methods used to treat lupus include methotrexate, antimalarial, cyclophosphamide, and antihormonal therapy as well as hormonal treatment. Antimalarial herbs are useful in treating lupus as one of the best Chinese herb therapies. According to traditional Chinese texts, summer heat causes red patches on the skin due to underlying heat toxin being activated in the blood.

These texts recommend the use of herbs to clear the heat and toxin or reducing the damp-heat impact. This could be due to sunlight, which is a primary trigger of this disease. These herbs then help in clearing heat and toxin that can bring this disease. Chinese-based medical journals were used in the 20th century all through the Ming dynasty era. This information source is still highly recognized.

In modern times, two major types of treating lupus with the use of selected herbs. This includes using antitoxin herbs alongside with ones that help with vitalizing blood circulation as well as ching-hao or its active components.

Since the use of Chinese literature on medical treatment of lupus is extensive, only a section of the information obtained from recent clinic-based trials is used in most articles to illustrate the type of use. However, discerning or representing the clinical results involving lupus can be difficult since the disease shows a high level of variability of manifestation on different patients over time.

The use of TCM has been used for years in the clinical setting to examine how different groups of people respond to the treatment. Some of the people involved in divisions include male and female, usually from various age groups. The units are then compared to each other with a difference in the disease ranging about three and half year's duration.

The group using herbs rely on types like Lingdan Pian, which includes moutan, ching-hao, Scrophularia chin-Chiu, buffalo horn, turtle shell and licorice among other herbs. In this test including the use of herbs alongside different type of remedies, the herbs showed significant results.

It is apparent that Chinese medicine has been in pursuit of using herbs in treating lupus for centuries. The good news is that herbs used in this type of medication are reliable and have proved useful in more than one instance.

Chapter 45
Remedies for Gout

G out is caused by a buildup of uric acid in the body and has been a severe problem for many people for quite some time. However, remember to avoid diet habits that could lead to inflammation problems, as this could lead to the development of gout. Perhaps the best part is that most of these treatments are not expensive, some of them are herbs you can grow in your lawn.

You can consume celery as seed extract or juice. The extract comes in handy when it comes to suppressing buildup of uric acid in your body. The herb comes with numerous benefits like antioxidants, from caffeine acid, phenolic acid, ferulic acid, and quercetin as well as flavanols. These properties make celery ideal for treating multiple conditions that can result from inflammation like joint pain, gout, infections in kidney or liver and skin disorders among others.

This alkaline mineral in magnesium has also been effective in treating gout by reducing the formation of uric acid in the body. Magnesium is effective in treating acute gout, and its deficiency in the body could lead to the development of gout. This means you should add magnesium supplements or foods rich in the mineral to your diet.

Proteolytic enzymes supplements come with bromelain, a potent remedy for gout. Bromelain is found mostly in a pineapple core. This is a digestive enzyme that has proved useful in suppressing inflammation and levels of uric acid in the body. This phenomenon explains why these proteins are a reliable solution for defeating gout and other serious problems.

Nettles herb is a potent anti-inflammatory phytonutrient that you can use as tea or supplementary drink. The anti-inflammatory properties in nettles are what make it a perfect solution for gout since the problem results from inflammation among other causes.

Fish oil may not produce instant effects, but with prolonged use, it helps decrease the risk of gout. This is all thanks to its high levels of omega-3 fatty acids that help in fighting inflammation, which can cause numerous diseases in your body. The use of this remedy helps fight gout and arthritis as well as other conditions that can result from inflammation.

The other remedy for gout is juice from black cherry or extract from cherry juice. This cherry comes with numerous benefits, with gout treatment being just one. According to studies being done, this remedy has shown potency to lower risk of gout with up to 35 percent. Besides, the use of this cherry can be used as a prescription for kidney stones as well.

Chapter 46
Herbs and Spices for a Healthy Heart

We use herbs and spices to enhance the taste and flavor of our foods all the time. But these spices can go beyond this to offer better health that we so desperately need.

Ginger comes with outstanding properties for blood thinning and inflammatory. The herb is also a helpful aid in digestion as well as treating nausea from motion sickness. You can get ginger by peeling and grating or chopping your ginger root and adding it to your soups, sauces, fruit, or vegetable drinks. Moreover, you can make tea from it or try it with honey.

Turmeric is handy in heart healing, with its curcumin compound helping with its healing potential. The herb is believed to be the secret behind low levels of Alzheimer's and arthritis in people who take it sufficiently. Curcumin is a potent anti-inflammatory and antioxidant compound for protection against cancer as well as boosting cardiovascular health. It also helps in preventing blood clot as well as lowering blood pressure and raising HDL cholesterol to healthy levels. Besides, a study has proven that the compound can inhibit enlargement of heart chambers. To get turmeric, just cook with the spice or curry.

Garlic has both antimicrobial and anti-inflammatory properties. Garlic was used to treat wounds, leprosy, infection, digestive disorders and cancer since time immemorial. Currently, the herb helps with cardiovascular health, thanks to its blood thinning properties. Besides, it offers unsurpassed efficiency in lowering blood cholesterol, pressure, and triglycerides as well as helping keep stomach, ovaries, and colon cancers at bay. Other benefits include fighting Borrelia, the Lyme causing bacteria.

Although cinnamon is considered as not so nutritious, it can be a great deal if you want to take control of your blood sugar through supporting the sensitivity of insulin. Besides, the herb comes with numerous antioxidant functions. If you are looking into boosting your blood's antioxidant levels, then this herb is one of the best options to try alongside rosemary, oregano, thyme, cloves and others. All you need to do is add it to your tea or sprinkle it on oatmeal.

Onion has almost similar benefits as garlic as the herbs come from the same family. Onions can lower blood pressure as well as reduce unhealthy fats in your blood. The herb also prevents clotting and reducing blood sugar. Onions are high in two antioxidant flavonoids, which are quercetin and sulfur. The former lowers blood pressure in hypertension patients. To get the best of onions, consider taking them raw, especially in salads or salsas.

Other herbs and spice that you need to get the best heart health include cayenne, capsaicin, cilantro, and rosemary. All of these herbs provide diverse benefits for your cardiovascular health as well as promoting health in other aspects of your body.

Chapter 47
Spices and Herbs for Weight Loss

Losing weight is one of the problems facing many people around the world, and a difficult one to overcome as well. Here are some of the best options to check out. Add only one teaspoon to your meals in a day, and cumin will help you burn up fat up to three times faster than you would in a day. The best part is that this spice is universal so that you can use it on virtually any type of food.

Cardamom spice is yet another thermogenic type, which works by helping the body temperature rise for better metabolism. It is best when mixed with cinnamon, nutmeg, ginger, and cloves when making a homemade chai tea or curry blend. Just like turmeric, or as you might have already learned, cayenne works by increasing body temperature and thus boosting metabolism. The spice can help in burning as much as 100 calories per meal. You can always sprinkle you cayenne over scrambled eggs, in soups, roasted nuts, or homemade dressings. Just be careful not to use much of it.

This bright yellow spice is known to help the body in burning fat. According to research, curcumin, an active compound in turmeric helps in losing fat efficiently. Overall, turmeric spice helps raise your body heat resulting in a higher metabolism. Turmeric also comes with several other benefits like fighting Alzheimer's disease and keeping hormones in check. You can add your turmeric to stews, soups or sprinkle it over roasted nuts or veggies.

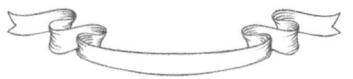

GARLIC MIGHT GIVE YOU bad breath, but its fat-burning benefits override the odds. Adding garlic to your meals is all you need to do, and it makes your food tastier as well. Black pepper not only helps in burning fat, but it is also efficient in blocking the formation of any new fat cells, which can help prevent weight gain altogether. Just add your black pepper to almost any food you are eating to get its benefits. The once considered just a weed; dandelion is winning the favor of many with its nutritional value and flavor in foods and drinks. The herb offers quite a good deal of weight loss as well as reducing bloat. Not forgetting, it is also efficient in increasing minerals as potassium and iron, as well as vitamin A, C, and E in your body. Cinnamon spice is useful in balancing blood sugar, thus keeping cravings under check. You can take it by sprinkling some on your oatmeal or mixing it in plain yogurt, cottage cheese, or any of your favorite brews for a bit more fragrance.

Chapter 48
Herbs and Roots for Healthier Liver

The liver is one of the most crucial organs in a person's body that is inevitable for survival. The liver performs significant functions in maintaining your overall health. From immunity to digestion, metabolism, and nutrient storage in the body, the lung provides numerous benefits for your health. Besides, this second largest organ in the body is a vital organ responsible for detoxification, providing nutrition and energy to tissues that might die without this necessary replenishment.

You can also keep your liver healthy by avoiding toxins that wear it down like alcohol, high fructose corn syrup, and acetaminophen. The other problem is HFCS, which has proved to cause liver scarring, which is common in cases of liver disease.

Turmeric's active component, curcumin, is rich in anti-inflammatory benefits that make it ideal for liver detoxing as well as ensuring general liver health. You can use the herb in your cooking or add it to your smoothie. Burdock root is used as the dandelion, but you might have to check with a local herbalist or online to find it. This herb is a potent blood purifier and further stimulates bile, which makes it a great option to go for if you want a healthier liver as well as overall blood health.

Milk thistle is also known as silibinin and is ideal for an herbal liver solution. You can use it as both a preventive measure against liver problems or for treating existing ones. If you want to add this herb to your diet, you can always count on its supplements to get the benefits that it offers.

Dandelion may be taken for just another yellow flower growing in your backyard, but it comes with numerous benefits for your body, and the liver is one of the organs that benefit the most. Dandelion is high in potassium, iron, and zinc. You need to use the herb and its roots to make the most of it. You can dig it out and use it to make tincture or tea.

The liver is essential for your overall health as it offers numerous benefits. From producing bile juice that aids in digestion to detoxifying the blood. Besides, it helps in getting rid of toxins and storing glucose as well as converting it to good sugar if the sugar levels in your blood drop below the recommended level. Among other benefits of the liver are the organs ability to break down hemoglobin and insulin as well as other hormones besides destroying worn-out red blood cells and converting ammonia to urea.

Maintaining your liver's health comes down to the type of lifestyle you embrace. This depends on different life factors like eating, exercise and reducing exposure to hazardous toxins that can destroy your liver. You can take advantage of numerous types of foods and liver-cleansing products, but these herbs are handy as well in keeping your liver in the best form possible and ensuring your body's immunity as well.

Chapter 49

Herbs and Spices to Fight Inflammation

We all like adding herbs and spices to our diet, perhaps to get the flavor or a better taste. But some herbs offer more than just the tantalizing flavor or the taste everyone is looking for; you can count on many health benefits that these herbs can provide. One of the things you will come to love about these herbs is the anti-inflammatory capabilities that you can count on to keep multiple diseases at bay.

Turmeric has been used in Indian medicine as well as Chinese medicine for years, treating arthritis, immune disorders, and liver disease among other problems. According to recent scientific studies, turmeric has proven to have antibacterial, antiviral, antifungal, anti-inflammatory, and anticancer properties among others. This makes the herb a viable option for treating arthritis, Alzheimer's disease, diabetes, allergies, as well as other chronic diseases.

These benefits come from the herb's compound curcumin, a potent antioxidant powerful enough to reduce inflammation. Besides, it is capable of inhibiting the development of tumor cells that cause different types of cancers. It is further useful in improving insulin resistance in most subjects through altering metabolic functions.

Cinnamon is known to reduce blood sugar levels in diabetic people by activating insulin receptors in the body. And like most other herbs, this one has many compounds high in antioxidants as well as anti-inflammatory properties, which are responsible for preventing cellular damage and the likelihood of chronic diseases.

Cloves contain a compound known as eugenol that is almost the same with cinnamon, only that this one is superior. Clove prevents inflammation, hence reducing chances of heart attack, cancer, as well as other chronic diseases. The spice works by inhibiting the COX-2 enzyme, which leads to inflammation. Not forgetting, it is also high in antioxidants.

Cayenne pepper has capsaicin, a compound useful for the spicy taste of cayenne as well as its medicinal properties. Cayenne is used in creams and ointments as a pain relief solution through depleting substance P in nerve cells, which is the chemical responsible for sending signals to the brain. This herb is potent with carotenoids, flavonoids, and antioxidants that help fight free radicals. This helps prevent cellular damage that leads to inflammation and subsequent diseases.

Ginger is another age-old remedy for pain and inflammation. It helps in soothing sore muscles, throat issues, as well as combating fatigue and aches. The spice attacks inflammation with the action of shogaols, gingerols, and paradols. Gingerol is a powerful antioxidant that prevents the production of free radicals known as peroxynitrite, which is responsible for causing inflammation and pain. Besides, these ginger compounds are used together to produce non-steroidal anti-inflammatory drugs.

If you are looking for an anti-inflammatory and antioxidant, then Rosemary is for you. It has compounds that help boost superoxide dismutase activity to remove the free radical superoxide, which is capable of causing chronic inflammation. Sage has carnosol and carnosic acids that help prevent inflammation that gives the herb its aroma. Besides, it improves memory and concentration, and its compounds have anticancer and antioxidant properties as well.

Chapter 50
Backyard Herbs with Medicinal Benefits

Whether you are fighting indigestion, pains, and aches or just about any other health problem, herbs are among the best natural remedies to try. But quite often, we tend to believe we can only get the best from a grocery store while leaving behind helpful weeds in our lawn. So what are some of the best options to try that you can find right in your backyard? Broadleaf plantain is nothing like the starchy banana tree plantain, but a small weed native of Asia and Europe. This plantain has been used in treating dysentery, toothaches, and reducing swelling. Moreover, its anti-inflammatory properties have also been used in cases of spider bites or bee stings.

Stinging Nettle is helpful in several ways and can be used in different forms as well. According to the USDA, you can use a cup of cooked Nettle to get your daily calcium needs and over a third of the required vitamin A and a significant amount of protein. All you need to do is remove the stinging hairs in this herb and boil it for a minute in two different glasses of water for each moment.

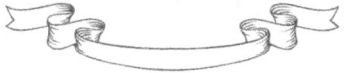

BURDOCK CAN PROVE DIFFICULT to control, but fun to enjoy. It makes a great option for a caffeine-free tea. The benefits are far-reaching too', as it has proved useful in controlling infections caused by topical fungal. Its roots also contain a compound to improve digestion, according to the University of Maryland medical center. Among the herbs that have been around for over a century, this one has its reasons for standing out. Self-Heal belongs to the mint family, and can be easily confused with a bugleweed, but its benefits are unmistakable. If you are looking for an antioxidant, then this herb is the one for you, which makes it a go-to option as a reliable medicinal herb.

Mullein comes with many names and benefits that have seen its extensive use in the West. Mullein is still useful for the modern day herbalists, thanks to its ability to treat numerous respiratory ailments. You can use it in tea to get the best of its juices that usually help with a sore throat and coughs. This herb can grow virtually anywhere, and it could be right in your backyard.

YOU CAN EASILY SPOT yarrow anytime in the early summer with its white-to-pink umbrella-like blossoms. Whether in your backyard, fields, or on the roadside, you can find it almost anywhere. This herb was useful o soldiers in WWI for soothing battered and bruised skin, but it also contains anti-inflammatory as well as antibacterial properties, which make it a powerful healing herb for different types of ailments. Dandelion bright yellow flowers make it stand out, and it grows almost anywhere. You can consume the leaves raw in sautés or salads, but you can also enjoy it in tea. The herb is high in beta-carotene and vitamin K, and it is helpful for cleansing liver and blood thanks to its perceived ability to stimulate the body to initiate a release of toxins.

Chapter 51
Preparing a Healthy Herbal Tea

A lmost everyone enjoys a cup of tea to start the day, perhaps to make the most of the disease-fighting, hydration or antioxidant effects that most teas offer. This might be the best option if you learn how to make a healthy beverage that can deliver more than just the kick you need for a morning boost. And there is no better way than making an herbal drink that comes with a pack of health benefits.

Well, a spoon of oolong, green, black or white tea could be a significant start to making a special tea that your family will enjoy. Such an herbal concoction is virtually all you need to keep your senses activated while still getting a great treat of the herbal goodness, but you can also try a caffeinated tea if you want to take things a step higher. Perhaps one of the things that make DIY tea blends a perfect choice is the fact that you can always prepare the tea that best matches your preference. Whether you want a different taste today, a dried option for yesterday may wait until another day, and you can always choose between the dehydrated, fresh, or a mixture of the two depending on your mood for the day.

A combination of base tea with some fresh herbs could go a long way, but for some, just a few leaves that are not teas could do the trick. For instance, a blend of holy basil, lemon balm, chamomile, and lavender can make an excellent concoction for relaxation. On the other end, a mix of rosemary, peppermint, lemon verbena and thyme will help soothe an illness. To pack your tea, you can pick a few teaspoons and put in a sachet or store in a jar to mix later; than you can store in an airtight jar for later use. However, make sure to use your fresh herbs for that day.

Make sure you know the measurement of the tea you want to prepare as well as the boiling drink, but remember to keep an eye on how long you boil it as well. For the dry types, boiling for fewer minutes goes a long way, but for the fresh leaves, you can let it cook longer. If you are making a blend of base teas and herb teas, stick to the instructions on the sachet. Once you have your tea brewed and ready, you can decide whether to let it cool down or dress it up for a better treat. A dollop of honey or steamed milk could add to the flavor and health of your tea, especially in case of yerba-based types. In case you are preparing iced tea, then you can add cups of cold water. Adding a few herbs into your glass can also help with flavor that your tea could offer.

Chapter 52
Soil for Better Herbs

G rowing herbs in your backyard can be fun, and a great way of using the time you are free, not to mention the rewards once the harvest time comes. And for every gardener, bringing out the best is always the most sought-after goal. Well, this could come down to the soil prepared for your herbs. You can create compost by decomposing vegetables and other organic material in a controlled chamber. You can always buy it in bags or prepare at home, depending on the amount that you need. However, it is important noting that commercial compost can vary significantly in quality.

When applying it in your garden, start by spreading about an inch or two over the growing bed, but the amount can vary depending on the soil quality, poor soil will require more. After applying the compost, you can use your shovel or fork to mix it with dirt, about six or nine inches or so. If you are looking for a replacement for the peat, then leaf mold is the better option. The best part about leaf mold is that you can prepare it in your backyard, but you will need about one deciduous tree and a bit of waiting to get it ready. To make the mold, use fresh leaves that have just fallen, put them in an enclosed box and wait. You don't have to balance the heat or turn it over with time, all you need to do is pile the leaves, and making sure to add moisture during dry periods, within a year, it will be ready.

Manure naturally comes from farm animals, apparently the cows and such. Make sure to keep your manure for about six months or so before applying it to your garden. You can decide to spread it over the open field, and then turn it in later or before your plant your herbs. But this can lead to the growth of weed from seeds in the manure. Besides, the slurry could contain unbroken herbicides from the way you raise the animals. But you can avoid such option and go for supply from someone who uses natural means to treat their animals and crops.

Peat moss offers an excellent conditioner for your soil. If you are working on sandy ground, it can add body, and for clay soil, it will help with lightening the soil texture. This moss includes plant material that has accumulated for years in areas known as peat lands. You can apply it in the garden before planting, but you need to be careful as it can acidify the soil. So you can consider using it on fields in the location you are planning to plant herbs that perform well in the acidic environment.

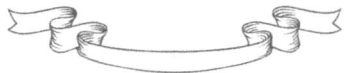

WORM CASTING ALSO KNOWN as vermicomposting, this option can be used for the same purpose as the compost to improve your soil's structure. Besides, this type can come in handy as a fertilizer that won't burn your plants, but be cautious and employ strategy on how you use it. If you are growing herbs such as thyme, hyssop, or borage, then the soil does not have to be too rich in nutrients, as this will mean the herbs will be less flavorful. But other types of calendula, lovage, and mint work better with more nutrients. So you can decide on the level of use depending on the herbs you are growing.

References

Brown AL, et al. Effects of Dietary Supplementation With the Green Tea Polyphenol Epigallocatechin-3-Gallate on Insulin Resistance and Associated Metabolic Risk Factors: Randomized Controlled Trial. British Journal of Nutrition. 2009 Mar;101(6):886-94. doi:10.1017/S0007114508047727.

https://draxe.com/

Hooper L, et al. Flavonoids, Flavonoid-Rich Foods, and Cardiovascular Risk: A Meta-Analysis of Randomized Controlled Trials. American Journal of Clinical Nutrition. 2008;88(1):38-50.

Kass L, Weekes J, Carpenter L. Effect of Magnesium Supplementation on Blood Pressure: A Meta-Analysis. European Journal of Clinical Nutrition. 2012;66(4):411-418.

Reinhart KM, Coleman CI, Teevan C, Vachhani P, White CM. Effects of Garlic on Blood Pressure in Patients With and Without Systolic Hypertension: A Meta-Analysis. Annals of Pharmacotherapy. 2008;42(12):1766-1771.

Ried K, Frank OR, Stocks NP, FaklerP, Sullivan T. Effect of Garlic on Blood Pressure: A Systematic Review and Meta-Analysis. BMC Cardiovascular Disorders. 2008;8:13.

Ried K, Sullivan TR, Fakler P, Frank OR, Stocks NP. Effect of Cocoa on Blood Pressure. The Cochrane Database of Systematic Reviews. 2012;8:CD008893.

Suzuki A, et al. Improvement of Hypertension and Vascular Dysfunction by Hydroxyhydroquinone-Free Coffee in a Genetic Model of Hypertension. FEBS Letters. 2006;580(9):2317-2322.t

132   ADIDAS WILSON

Wahabi HA, Alansary LA, Al-Sabban AH, Glasziuo P. The Effectiveness of Hibiscus Sabdariffa in the Treatment of Hypertension: A Systematic Review. Phytomedicine. 2010;17(2):83-86.

Fan Yongsheng, et al, Observation on clinical effect of hormone combined with toxin-cleaning, stasis-resolving, and yin-nourishing method for the treatment of systemic lupus erythematosus, Chinese Journal of Integrated Traditional Chinese Medicine and Western Medicine 1999; 19(10): 626-627.

Wen Chengping, et al, Effect of Langchuangding on serum soluble interleukin-2 receptor and neopterin level in patients of systemic lupus erythematosus, Chinese Journal of Integrated Traditional Chinese Medicine and Western Medicine 2001; 21(5): 339-341.

Zhong Jiaxi, et al, 25 cases of systemic lupus erythematosus treated by integrated traditional Chinese medicine and Western medicine, Chinese Journal of Integrated Traditional Chinese Medicine and Western Medicine 1999; 19(1): 47-48.

Wu Xiang, et al, Clinical observation on nephrotic syndrome of lupus nephritis treated with integrated Chinese and Western medicine, Chinese Journal of Integrated Traditional Chinese Medicine and Western Medicine 1998; 18(12): 718-720.

Wang ZY, Clinical and laboratory studies of the effect of an antilupus pill on systemic lupus erythematosus, Chinese Journal of Integrated Traditional Chinese Medicine and Western Medicine 1989; 9(8): 465-468, 452.

Auerbach, P. Auerbach: Wilderness Medicine. 5th ed. Philadelphia, PA: Elsevier Mosby; 2007.

Bradley P, ed. British Herbal Compendium. Vol. I. Dorset (Great Britain): British Herbal Medicine Association; 1992:149-150.

Brinker F. Herb Contraindications and Drug Interactions. 3rd ed. Sandy, OR: Eclectic Medical Publications; 2001:93-94.

Davison GC, Rosen RC. Lobeline and reduction of cigarette smoking. Psychol Rep. 1972;31:443-56.

Dwoskin LP, Crooks PA. A novel mechanism of action and potential use for lobeline as a treatment for psychostimulant abuse. Biochem Pharmacol. 2002;63(2):89-98.

Han SR, Lv XY, Wang YM, et al. A study on the effect of aqueous extract of Lobelia chinensis on colon precancerous lesions in rats. Afr J Tradit Complement Altern Med. 2013;10(6):422-5.

Karch SB. The Consumer's Guide to Herbal Medicine. Hauppauge, NY: Advanced Research Press; 1999:127-128.

Kuo YC, Lee YC, Leu YL, Tsai WJ, Chang SC. Efficacy of orally administered Lobelia chinensis extracts on herpes simplex virus type 1 infection in BALB/c mice. Antiviral Res. 2008;80(2):206-12.

Lim DY, Kim YS, Miwa S. Influence of lobeline on catecholamine release from the isolated perfused rat adrenal gland. Auton Neurosci. 2004;110(1):27-35.

Marlow SP, Stoller JK. Smoking cessation. Respir Care. Dec 2003;48(12):1238-54; discussion 1254-6.

Mazur LJ, De Ybarrondo L, Miller J, Colasurdo G. Use of alternative and complementary therapies for pediatric asthma. Tex Med. 2001;97(6):64-68.

Newall C, Anderson L, Phillipson J. Herbal Medicines: A Guide for Health-care Professionals. London: Pharmaceutical Press; 1996:187.

Rotblatt M, Ziment I. Evidence-Based Herbal Medicine. Philadelphia, PA: Hanley & Belfus, Inc; 2002:259-261.

Stead LF, Hughes JR. Lobeline for smoking cessation (Cochrane Review). In: The Cochrane Library, 1, 2002. Oxford: Update Software.

Subarnas A, Tadano T, Oshima Y, Kisara K, Ohizumi Y. Pharmacological properties of beta-amyrin palmitate, a novel centrally acting compound, isolated from Lobelia inflata leaves. J Pharm Pharmacol. 1993;45(ISS 6):545-550.

Subarnas A, Tadano T, Nakahata N, et al., A possible mechanism of antidepressant activity of beta-amyrin palmitate isolated from

Lobelia inflata leaves in the forced swimming test. Life Sci. 1993;52(3):289-96.

Subarnas A, Oshima Y, Sidik, Ohizumi Y. An antidepressant principle of Lobelia inflata L. (Campanulaceae). J Pharm Sci. 1992;53(7):620-621.

Wilhelm CJ, Johnson RA, Eshleman AJ, Janowsky A. Lobeline effects on tonic and methamphetamine-induced dopamine release. Biochem Pharmacol. Mar 15 2008;75(6):1411-5.

Aboelsoud, N.H. (2010). Herbal Medicine in Ancient Egypt, Journal of Medicinal Plants Research, 4(2), 82-86, 18 January, DOI: 10.5897/JMPR09.013

Ede, A. & Cormack, L.B. (2012). A History of Science in Society: From the Ancient Greeks to the Scientific Revolution, North York, Ontario, Canada: University of Toronto Press

Jouanna, J. (2012). Greek Medicine from Hippocrates to Galen: Selected Papers, Leiden, The Netherlands: Koninklijke Brill

Mininberg, D.T. (2005). The Legacy of Ancient Egyptian Medicine. In J.P. Allen (Ed.). The Art of Medicine in Ancient Egypt, New York, Metropolitan Museum Press: 13-15

Nunn, J.F. (1996). Ancient Egyptian Medicine, Norman, OK: University of Oklahoma Press

Teichberg S, Wingertzahn MA, Moyse J, Wapnir RA. Effect of gum arabic in an oral rehydration solution on recovery from diarrhea in rats. J Pediatr Gastroenterol Nutr. 1999 Oct;29(4):411-7.

Schütz K, Carle R, Schieber A. Taraxacum–a review on its phytochemical and pharmacological profile. J Ethnopharmacol. 2006 Oct 11;107(3):313-23. Epub 2006 Jul 22. Review.

Saller R, Melzer J, Reichling J, Brignoli R, Meier R. An updated systematic review of the pharmacology of silymarin. Forsch Komplementmed. 2007 Apr;14(2):70-80. Epub 2007 Apr 23. Review.

Aga M, Iwaki K, Ueda Y, Ushio S, Masaki N, Fukuda S, Kimoto T, Ikeda M, Kurimoto M. Preventive effect of Coriandrum sativum

(Chinese parsley) on localized lead deposition in ICR mice. J Ethnopharmacol. 2001 Oct;77(2-3):203-8.

Shkurupiĭ VA, Kazarinova NV, Ogirenko AP, Nikonov SD, Tkachev AV, Tkachenko KG. [Efficiency of the use of peppermint (Mentha piperita L) essential oil inhalations in the combined multi-drug therapy for pulmonary tuberculosis]. Probl Tuberk. 2002;(4):36-9. Russian.

Testai L, Chericoni S, Calderone V, Nencioni G, Nieri P, Morelli I, Martinotti E. Cardiovascular effects of Urtica dioica L. (Urticaceae) roots extracts: in vitro and in vivo pharmacological studies. J Ethnopharmacol. 2002 Jun;81(1):105-9.

†Results may vary. Information and statements made are for education purposes and are not intended to replace the advice of your doctor. Adidas Wilson does not dispense medical advice, prescribe, or diagnose illness. The views and nutritional advice expressed by Adidas Wilson are not intended to be a substitute for conventional medical service. If you have a severe medical condition or health concern, see your physician.